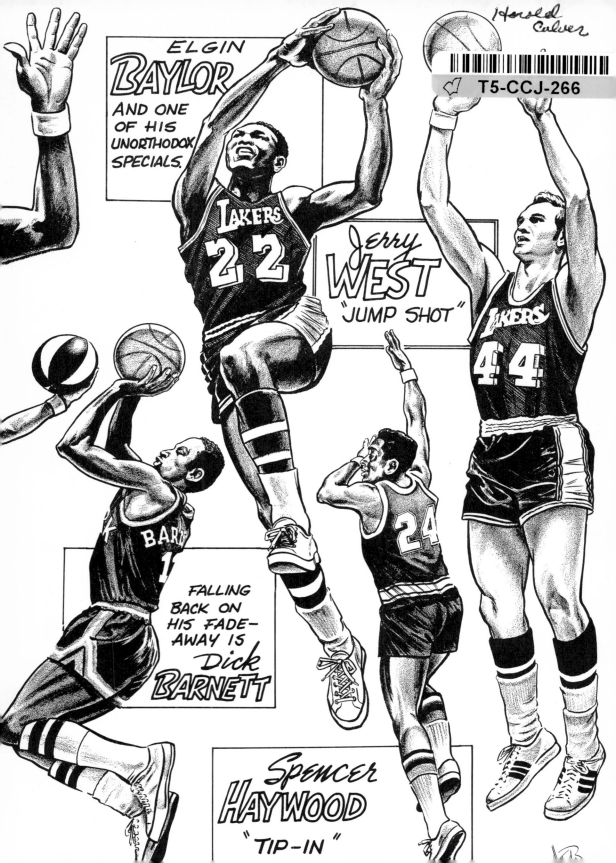

Basketball My Way

by
JERRY WEST
with
BILL LIBBY

PRENTICE-HALL, INC.

Englewood Cliffs, N.J.

Basketball My Way by Jerry West and Bill Libby

Copyright © 1973 by Jerry West and Bill Libby
Drawings copyright © 1973 by Art Brewster

Printed in the United States of America

Prentice-Hall International, Inc., London
Prentice-Hall of Australia, Pty. Ltd., North Sydney
Prentice-Hall of Canada, Ltd., Toronto
Prentice-Hall of India Private Ltd., New Delhi
Prentice-Hall of Japan, Inc., Tokyo

Library of Congress Cataloging in Publication Data

West, Jerry
Basketball my way.

SUMMARY: Discusses the objectives of basketball
and techniques of playing the game.
1. Basketball—Juvenile literature. [1. Basketball]
I. Libby, Bill, joint author. II. Title.
GV885.1.W48   796.32'3   72-7064
ISBN 0-13-072439-4

10 9 8 7 6 5 4 3 2

*For my sons
David, Mark, and Michael.
May they enjoy playing this game,
whether for pleasure
or a profession.*

JERRY WEST

ACKNOWLEDGMENTS   The cover photo and most other photos in this book were taken by Wen Roberts and other staff photographers of Johnny Johnson's Photography, Inc., 325 E. Florence Avenue, Inglewood, California.

Many photos were taken from an instructional film prepared for distribution by Sunkist Growers, Inc., with permission secured through Rene Henry, Jr., Publicity, 340 19th St., Santa Monica, California.

Other photos were secured through the Los Angeles Lakers and other teams in the National Basketball Association and American Basketball Association, and Sears, Roebuck and Company, sponsors of Laker basketball clinics, through the courtesy of T. A. Santo.

All drawings are by Art Brewster, 5681 Abraham Street, Westminster, California.

The authors also wish to thank Robert Gerst, Fred Schaus, Dr. Robert Kerlan, Frank O'Neill, Jim Brochu, Stu Zanville, Bill Sharman, Jim McMillian, Chuck Montero, Kevin Hawkins, and many other persons, including players and team publicists, for making this book possible.

Contents

1. The Game

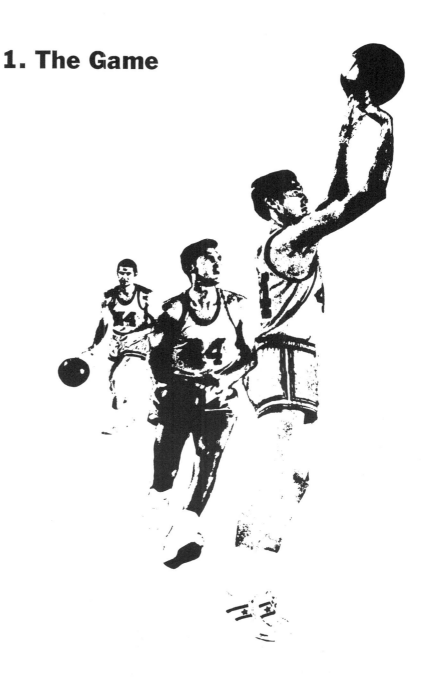

My jump shot—in sequence. (William East-abrook for Sunkist Growers)

THE GAME of basketball is both an individual and a team game. It is an individual game first, but it is a team game in the end. The individual's play must be meshed into team play. I am one of those who sincerely believes it matters a lot less how the player does than how the team does. Thus many of the things I say in this book will be directed toward making the player a better team player.

This will help the player more than he may realize because the better team player he is, the further he is likely to go in the game. However, I am less concerned with helping a few players who will go all the way to the pros than I am with helping many players do better and thus get more pleasure out of the game however far they go.

Actually, the fundamentals a player uses and his approach to the game should be the same on all levels. Hopefully, this book will be helpful to all, from beginners to accomplished players.

One of the beauties of basketball is that a player can practice a lot by himself. A football player can pass for accuracy and punt for accuracy and distance by himself, but it is difficult for him to perfect his passing if he isn't throwing to a moving target, it is difficult for him to

THE GAME, at the start, the center-jump from overhead at the Forum in the Los Angeles suburb of Inglewood, where my Lakers play their home games. Here, Wilt Chamberlain, right, is jumping against Jim Fox, then of Phoenix. I'm at the upper right with a hand out to keep track of Dick Van Arsdale. (Photography, Inc.)

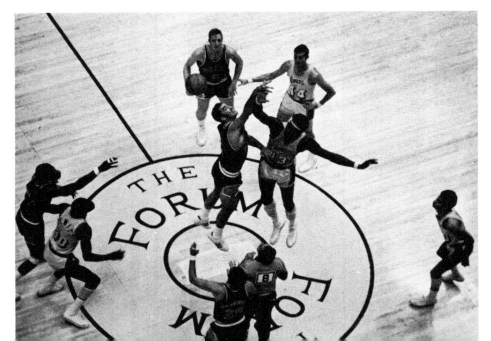

place-kick without a holder, it is impossible for him to
develop running skills without tacklers to avoid. A baseball player can practice pitching against a wall, but it is
difficult to develop without a catcher and batter, it is
impossible to develop batting skills without a pitcher,
and it is impossible to develop fielding skills without
someone to hit the ball.

A basketball player can develop different shots and
shootings skills, rebounding and dribbling abilities, all by
himself to a great degree. I know because I did. As a boy
growing up in Cheylan, West Virginia, I was alone a lot. I
spent much time playing by myself on a dirt court with
a basket and backboard a neighbor had in his backyard.

Television was just beginning when I was a boy, and I
did not get to see all the great stars of all sports the way
my three sons do today. Pro football and pro basketball
weren't very big in those days, at least not around West
Virginia. I followed the high school and college games on
the radio.

I remember the times I got to go to West Virginia
University basketball games. We sat way high and the
court seemed very far away and the players seemed very
small, but I was really thrilled. I can remember imagining
myself playing down there on the court some day,
though I was so small I don't think I really believed it
ever could happen. I'd go home and imitate all the different players, imagining I was them, practicing on that
neighbor's court all by myself. When I started on that
court, I was so small and the ball so heavy that I had to
shoot two-handed and underhanded with all my might
just to reach the basket.

Basketball is basically a simple game, and I am not
going to make it appear confusing by using a lot of com-
plex instructions in this book. I am not going to throw a
lot of charts and diagrams at the reader. I am using a lot
of posed-for pictures to illustrate particular points and
unposed pictures of the great stars of the game to show
how they look in action.

My way of playing this game is not the way all other

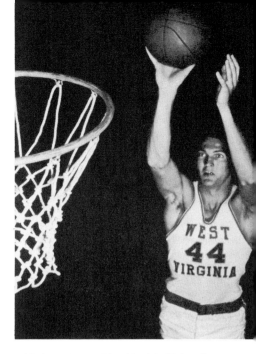

My jumpshot at West Virginia University.

As a pro I drive against the bearded Wally
Jones, then with the Philadelphia 76ers.
(Photography, Inc.)

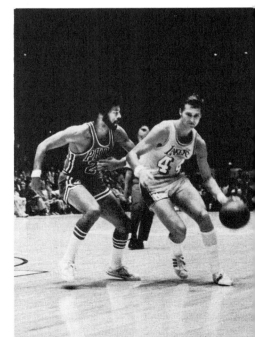

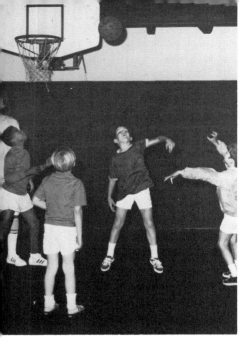

The younger element is shown in these pictures. Above, I watch as my three sons join Tom Hawkins' son, directly in front of me, in a scrimmage in front of our garage. That's Michael shooting over David while Mark watches. Below, Pasadena and East Pasadena boys' club teams mix it up between halves of a pro game at the Forum. (Photography, Inc.)

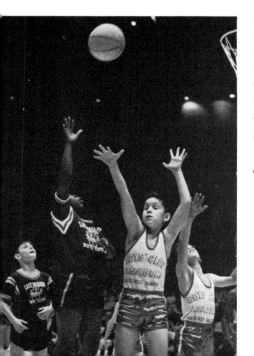

players play it. My way of teaching it is to point out the various ways various things can be done effectively. The reader will see the different ways different players do things and, hopefully, will look for certain things when they watch the stars.

I believe the most important way to play the game is the way it comes most naturally to you, but you must have a solid base on which to build your finished form. Every player's style can be improved so that it brings out the most of his abilities. Good players do many things differently, but, beneath the style that shows on the surface, we use similar fundamentals.

I am a guard, but I played forward in high school and college and I've been around centers long enough to know something of pivot play. While describing the ways to do things, I'll keep it in mind that some things have to be done differently depending on the position a player plays, but players may change positions from time to time, and I believe it is important to be a well-rounded player, so I suspect all players can be helped by all areas of instruction.

Since most players are right-handed, the instruction in this book is written for right-handers, but left-handers should be able to reverse certain details and be equally benefited by it.

I am small as pro players go, at 6-3 and 185 pounds, but I believe the basics are the same whether a player is 5-4 or 7-4. It is clear the 5-4 player should be more concerned with backcourt play, while the 7-4 player should be more concerned with pivot play, but it is not clear that height alone should determine a player's best position. As he is developing, the player should not ignore the needs of players in other positions or ignore the possibility that he may switch positions in time.

When I was eleven or twelve I was only about 5-6 and didn't even weigh 100 pounds. I was so small the other

kids wouldn't let me play football with them and I'd
wind up back on my basketball court. Actually, football
was my first love, but when I tried out for my junior
high school team I was so small they didn't have a uniform to fit me, and I wound up as the team manager. I
love baseball and played some sandlot ball, but we didn't
have Little League or other organized baseball leagues.
Basketball was big in West Virginia and I got sidetracked
into that and found out it was best for me. It took a
while to figure that out. I wasn't very good at first. As a
seventh-grader I only got to dress for one or two games.

The point I am making is that it doesn't matter how
small you are or whether you think you are good enough
to play basketball. If you learn to play as best you can
you never know how you will develop later. Small players play effectively in high school and college ball, and
even sometimes in pro ball. I think 5-9 Calvin Murphy's
play in pro basketball is going to create many more opportunities for small men. And the longer I am in basketball the more I am amazed at how many good players in
grade school or high school or college fail to become
good players on the next level and how many ordinary
players on every level develop into stars.

I was not a starter for my East Bank High School
team at first. Even after becoming an all-American at
West Virginia University, I was not a starter for the Los
Angeles Lakers when I first went into pro basketball. Yet
I have made some all-time All-Star basketball teams,
have led the NBA in scoring, have led the NBA in assists,
and have been voted to All-Star defensive teams. I would
never have guessed I would do anything like it when I
was a boy.

The point here is: don't get discouraged. If you want
it enough, do your best and wait for the best in you to
come out. Learn what you're doing from the ground up.
Building a basketball player is like building anything

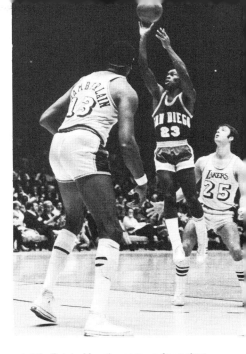

Little Calvin Murphy goes up for a shot
flanked by another successful small man,
Gail Goodrich, and a rather big man, Wilt
Chamberlain. (Photography, Inc.)

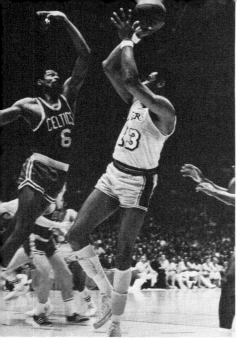

Classic confrontations of Wilt Chamberlain against major rivals are shown in these Wen Roberts photos. Above, Boston's Bill Russell goes up to attempt to block Wilt's shot.

Milwaukee's Kareem Abdul-Jabbar fronts Wilt as they await developments in an especially graphic depiction of intense concentration. (Photography, Inc.)

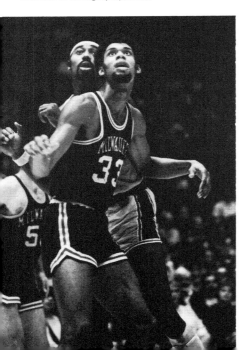

else—you start with the foundation. If the foundation is solid, the rest will be more solid. I don't say a natural athlete can't pick up what he needs later, but I think it gets harder as you go along.

The player starts with a lot of practice by himself. Then he practices with others, playing a lot of pickup games. Eventually, teams are formed or he gets into an organized league. I'll cover these steps as we go along. And in the end I'll stress team play.

I shall give fundamental tips and more advanced suggestions in this book. Some of what I suggest may be helpful to coaches. And while I believe a player should do what his coach wants him to do, I am not going to pretend that coaches are always right. Some players are hurt by their coaches. But I believe that in the long run it is important for a player to accept his coach's advice and perform as part of a team, because then the team will be most likely to win games.

Some players will be played out of their best positions because it helps the team and if you aren't willing to do this, then turn to something else. Most players are helped by most coaches. Most coaches have played the game and understand it and have given their lives to it, so it is foolish for the young player to feel he knows more. In the long run the player who works hard at doing what he is asked to do will go the furthest. Allowing unhappiness with some situation to affect their play has hurt many players.

Over the years I have observed that players tend to blame all their problems on the coach. For this reason I have reservations about ever becoming a coach. I don't know if I could coach knowing the way players are bound to talk about me behind my back.

The fact is, coaches make mistakes, but most coaches use their best players the best way they can and pick their regulars on the basis of what they can do on the court and not on their personalities. They do this because they want to win. It is that simple.

Some coaches are better than others. Some are strong in some areas and weak in others. Some are good at fundamentals, others at preparing for an opponent, still others at running a game. Some have the sort of personality that reaches people, that makes them loved; others are demanding types. The fact is, good players can win with any coach if they do what he asks them to do, if they play the same game and pull together.

I've liked and respected all of my coaches, though in different ways, from the very beginning. Duke Shaver was my basketball coach at Cheylan Junior High School. He was a fine man, inspirational to the players, and a good coach, very strong on conditioning. As a kid I liked to goof off, but the stress he put on an athlete staying in shape stuck with me. It's not unusual for a boy to be inclined to clown around. The sooner you get serious, however, the faster you'll improve. Just playing the game should be fun enough.

The basketball coach at East Bank High School was Roy Williams. He was an exceptional coach, in some ways the best I ever had. There is no reason to look down on your coach in junior high school or high school because he's not a big name or a pro. Many are capable of coaching on any level. They either didn't get a break or didn't seek it. Roy Williams stressed fundamentals, defense and team play. Under his guidance I first began to become a well-rounded player.

In college and again in the first part of my professional career, my coach was Fred Schaus. He has a brilliant basketball mind and prepared our teams for the teams and games we had to play as well as any man I've ever known. We always went into our games feeling we were ready. That is a very big thing. Some coaches are not well-organized and waste a lot of time between games.

Bill van Breda Kolff was one of the most determined men I've ever known. He didn't get as technical as some coaches, but he filled you with a lot of desire. Guys really want to play for Bill. This also is a very big thing.

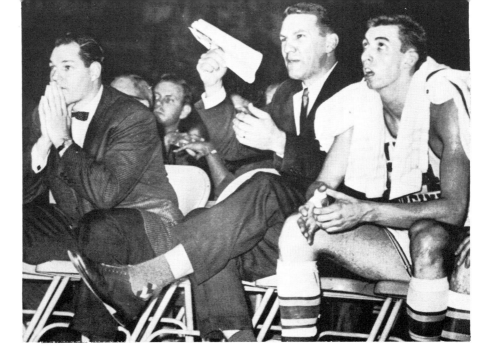

Fred Schaus (center), my coach at West Virginia University and later with the Lakers, then general manager of the Lakers. (Photography, Inc.)

It's fun playing for Bill, but it doesn't stop you from wanting to win. Winning is the most fun I know.

Joe Mullaney was a very nice guy, very low-keyed and very imaginative. He tried a lot of different things and brought some new ideas to the pro game. I felt bad when he got fired. This is the business. We didn't win the championship, but only one team wins the championship every season, and it can be a cruel business where coaches are concerned. I think young players should realize that there is a great deal of pressure on their coaches at every level, that in the end they are dependent on a lot of guys running around in their underwear doing a job. The more you play, the more sympathetic you become to a coach's problems.

Bill Sharman is a coach I've always admired. Teams always seem to do better under him than they do under other coaches. He's a nice, understanding, soft-spoken man off the court, but a very tough man on it. He is intense and demands concentration at all times and works his players exceptionally hard in practice. He is tremendously well-organized and devoted to details. He feels many games every season and many championships often turn on getting the loose ball, getting the big rebound, making the right play in the right spot, and I think he is right. Although we had some older players, including Wilt and myself, he prefers a running style and sold us on a running game and it paid off.

He made us so much of a team with not only all five players on court at a time but many members off our bench contributing that it was the easiest season I've had in many seasons and gave me a new lease on life. Under him, we set an all-time pro record for sports teams with 33 straight victories, won more games, 69, than any team in pro history, lost only 13, and finally won the elusive NBA title in 1972 after dethroning a Milwaukee team that was supposed to be on a dynasty. His players improve under him, team play improves under him and his teams win.

This game means a lot to him, so he gives it everything he has. It means more to some than to others. I can't tell you how much it should mean to you, but I think the more it means the better you will do. Talent alone will carry a guy only so far. I have always been very intense, get very nervous before games, am very emotional during games and feel pretty washed-out after games. I really wouldn't wish this on anyone. I'm never satisfied. No matter what worked for me, I'm always

An intense coach, Bill Sharman, right, watches action from the sidelines.

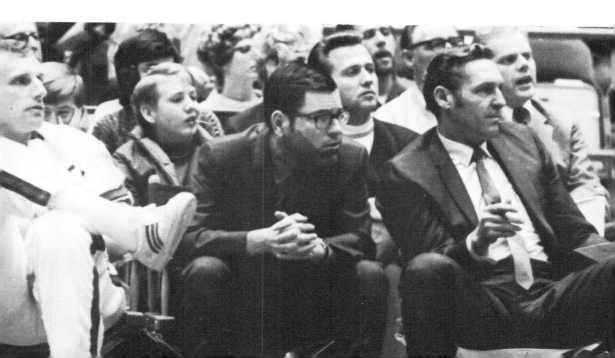

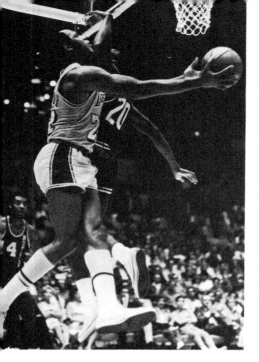

Elgin Baylor, always cool and calm, even when getting an elbow in the jaw, shoots a typical Elgin Baylor shot, two-handed, underhanded, from behind the backboard and almost directly under the basket. That's Oscar Robertson watching at the left. (Photography, Inc.)

thinking of all the mistakes I made and the chances I missed. Players should aim at perfection. No one will reach it. Few will come close. But if you don't try for it, you won't ever come close.

Some fellows don't show tension as much as others. Elgin Baylor could be joking around five seconds before we took the court and ten seconds before the opening tipoff, but when the game began he got deadly serious. It was his personality. Never did Elg give less than his best in games. This is a cliché, but it's true of Elg. I've known many who gave much less than their best. It just doesn't mean that much to them. They should be doing something else.

Hot Rod Hundley is a good friend of mine, though we're different personalities. Life is a party for Rod. He can't seem to take anything seriously. He was a great high school player and a college all-American at West Virginia. He was the first draft choice of the entire NBA. But he seldom played regularly and lasted only six years in pro ball. When he found out it didn't come easy to him on this level and he'd have to work at it, he couldn't bring himself to do it. He'd never done it before. Suddenly he was gone from the game. Today he broadcasts games, but I think he misses playing it and regrets he didn't become better at it. His life is unsettled and he never knows what he's going to do from year to year. That's his way of life. He seems happy. Everyone loves him, but I think he's wasted a lot of himself. You have to decide which way you want to go.

I think a player should make up his mind that if he is going to play this game at all he is going to play it right; that while he is playing it he is going to concentrate on it. He is not going to be thinking about Friday night's party or Saturday night's date or Sunday's movie. It is time enough to think about these things when they come along. I feel a fellow should live for today, for right now. Yesterday is gone, tomorrow may never come. The only thing we can control is what's happening right now.

The player should buy a rule book and read it and reread it and learn it and keep referring to it. The basic rules are simple. The degree of permissible contact varies from area to area and level to level. Five fouls put you out of high school and college games, six fouls put you out of pro games. High school games last 32 minutes, college games 40 minutes, pro games 48 minutes. The player has to understand the game he's playing, the limitations under which he plays. The rule book is the best place to begin. Close observation is another. Playing still another. But by the time you begin to play, you should know the rules.

I'll be talking in this book of the game of basketball not as it was designed but as it is played. It was designed as a noncontact game. It has become a contact game. The higher you go the more contact is permitted. The court is small and the higher you go the bigger the players get. Ten players in tight quarters are going after one ball and one basket at each end of the court. It gets rough out there. That's the way it is. I'll try to help the player prepare for it.

It is a game that is controlled by the officials. The referees play a critical part in every game. There are a lot of fouls called and a lot of free throws awarded in most games, and many games are decided by this. Again, this is the way it is. It destroys a player's concentration if he constantly yells at the referees, and it rarely gets him anywhere.

Referees make mistakes. Players make mistakes, too. There is not a harder game to officiate than basketball. You have to remember this. Most referees are doing an enormously difficult job as best they can, and most are very good. They're off to the side, in a better position to see what happens than the player caught up in the middle of the action. I get steamed at refs a lot, and it's not

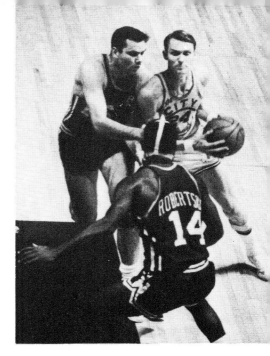

The American Basketball Association has produced some fine basketball since its formation. One of its brightest stars in its early years has been Rick Barry (above) with San Francisco of the NBA before jumping to the ABA, driving against the defense of one superstar, Jerry Lucas, into another, Oscar Robertson, who is wearing a mask to protect an injury. Below, Zelmo Beaty (31) a fine center, goes for a rebound for the Utah Stars, the team Bill Sharman coached to the ABA playoff title in 1971. (Paul Barker, Deseret *News*.)

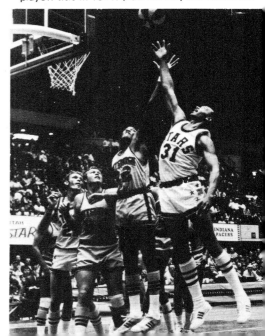

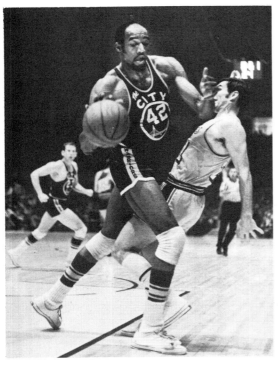
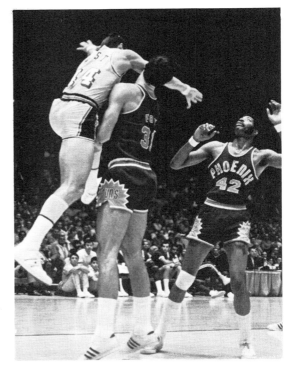
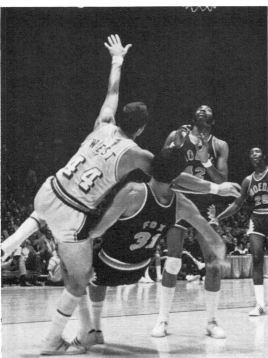
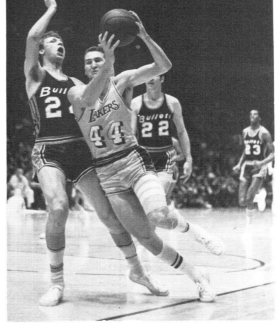

Rough and rugged play is a part of basketball these days. Top left, big and brilliant center Nate Thurmond barges right through me. I seem to be feeling it, too. However, I do some barging of my own (top right) as I arrive too late to block a shot by Connie Hawkins (42) and in my anxiety bowl over Jim Fox (bottom left). My leg bandaged to protect an injury (bottom right), I drive on a Baltimore Bullet, who seems to be saying something in protest of my enthusiasm. (Photography, Inc.)

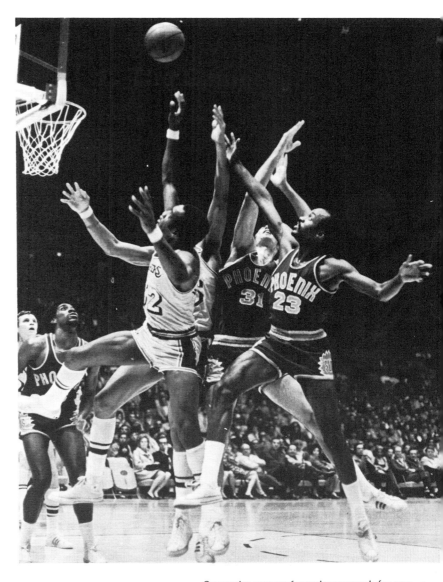

Count the arms as four players reach for one ball in this classic shot of action in a Los Angeles-Phoenix game. I can pick out Happy Hairston (52), Mel Counts (31), and Art Harris (23.) (Photography, Inc.)

good. But I seldom say anything to them. The main thing is just to put resentment aside and turn to the next play.

The big play in basketball is the shot that goes in, the score. You win by scoring more than the other team. But you also win by holding the other team to less

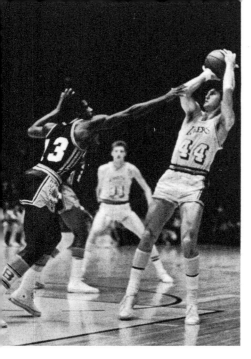

Under fierce pressure applied on defense by a Baltimore player, I draw back in an attempt to shoot over him and, being off-balance, probably missed the shot. (Photography, Inc.)

Driving for a two-hand underhand shot in close, I prepare to lay the ball over leaping defender Lou Hudson. Walt Hazzard is watching at the right. (Photography, Inc.)

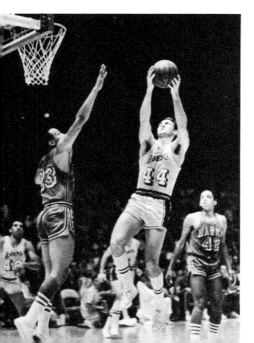

points than you get. I think defense wins more games than offense. I'm prouder of my defense than I am of my offense. Kids usually concentrate on shooting. As you reach the top level, great shooters are a dime a dozen. The players who can get loose for good shots are a lot rarer. The players who can take the good shots away from the best shooters are rare. The players who can make the best plays and break up the best plays are rare. More players can play good offense than can play good defense. Thus the better defensive players turn games around more than the better offensive players.

You pick up the paper the day after a game and you read that such-and-such a team won because so-and-so scored 30 points. It's just as likely this team won because some other player set the scorer up with some passes or because still another player took three or four baskets away from the other team's best scorer. It's hard to stop a great scorer completely, but if you take two or three or four baskets away from him, that may be the difference between winning and losing. The turning point in a game may be the blocked shot or the steal or the deflected pass at the key moment, though this seldom is written about and is hidden beneath the surface. After you play the game awhile, though, you know. You come to know what is most important.

I'm a scorer. Usually, I have to shoot well if I'm going to help my team win. But I can do other things, such as make good plays and play defense. If I'm not shooting well, I do more of those other things. The other things aren't what made me famous, but that doesn't make them any less important. You have to do a lot of things that aren't noticed. The coach and the other players will usually notice. And even if they don't, you will know. You have to accept the fact that most people don't play this game and don't come to know it as players do. You have to rely a lot on personal pride.

I'm as proud of having made a number of all-star defensive teams in the NBA in recent seasons as I am of having made the regular all-star teams over the years. I'm as proud of having led the NBA in assists during the 1971-72 season as I was of having led it in scoring during the 1969-70 season. Bill Sharman developed a style of team play with the Lakers that did not depend as much on my scoring as previous Laker teams had. I still averaged 25 points a game. But Gail Goodrich averaged 25 points, too, And I averaged more than nine assists a game, which translates to 18 points a game. Wilt Chamberlain, the greatest scorer the game has known, averaged less than 15 points a game, but led the league with more than 19 rebounds a game, triggered our fast-breaks and played tremendous defense. A player has to give what the team needs from him. There are a lot of ways to play this game, and you play the way that wins for your team. When I suffered a severe shooting slump in the 1972 playoffs, I still had other things to contribute to my team.

The player should take instruction and practice seriously. We all have a tendency to think we know it all. But I have never stopped learning and I don't think any good player ever has. My thinking has changed a lot over the years. I'm not the same player or person I was ten or fifteen years ago, or even last year. I don't think anyone ever is. We don't think we'll change, but we do. Keep this in mind. Be flexible and open to change.

Work for consistency. The more I play the game, the more I become convinced it is the most important thing a player can bring to the court. If the other players and the coach know what they can count on from the player, his value is at its highest. I'd rather be the kind of player who scores 20 points three games in a row than the player who scores 40 in one game and ten in the next and 20 in the next. I'd rather do an all-around job

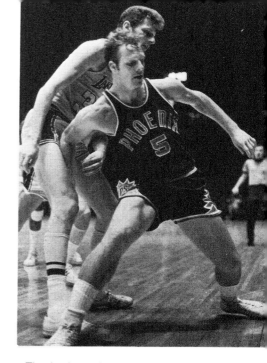

The shoving and pushing for position in close is not a simple thing for a distant ref to pass judgment on. Here Dick Van Arsdale, not a super-scorer but one of the toughest and most consistent players in pro ball, blocks out big Mel Counts.

every game than sluff off on defense to score high in some games.

The player should play hard in every game, during every play of every game. It is not an easy thing to do. Things go wrong and we get discouraged. Things go right and we get overconfident. Sooner or later we get tired. Maybe things other than basketball are bothering us. But the player is only going to be with the game a few hours at a time, and it is really not so much to ask that he bear down and give it everything he has. The player who makes a habit of going all-out will go further. Sheer hustle can make up for a lot of flaws.

You build a solid base and build on it, both mentally and physically. You can't start at the top. You have to get there. Some get there sooner than others, but some with less talent will make it where others with more talent will not because some try hader and build a sounder base.

The college game certainly is a spectacular one with superstars on their way up, so I see as many games on this level as I can. Here, in one of the classic games of the 1970-71 season, Austin Carr of Notre Dame, an all-American and later the first choice in the pro draft, shoots over Curtis Rowe of UCLA, another all-American and a high draft-pick, as the host Irish handed the Bruins their only defeat of the season enroute to another national championship. (Jim Hunt)

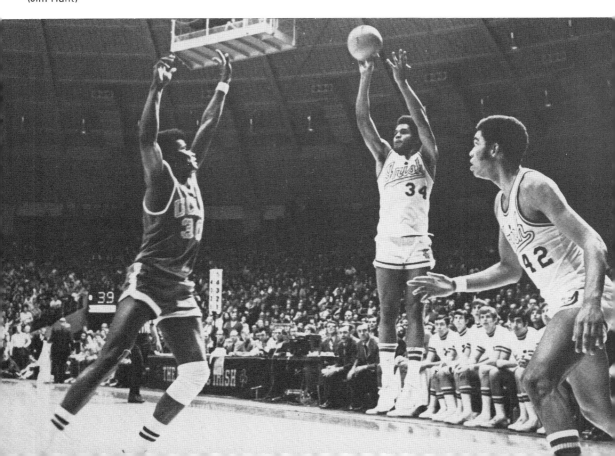

I am somewhat embarrassed by my nickname, "Mr. Clutch," which is the title of my biography, because I am not by nature a vain person, though I am a proud person. And I am proud of the nickname, because it indicates that I have come through many times under pressure. A lot of players lose their poise under pressure. I will try to explain how players can overcome this. A player should do his best when it counts the most.

I've been injury-prone and have been sidelined more than most players. But I've also often played with injuries. A good player can't play in fear of getting hurt. Accidents happen, but there are things a player can do to avoid many injuries and to come back as strong as possible from those he does suffer. I'll try to indicate how I think you should handle yourself off the court to help you do your best on the court.

I've played on teams that won many pennants and divisional championships in pro ball. I've played on a team that won a state high school championship. I've also played on a team that lost the national college title by 1 point in the last game. And I've played on teams that prior to the 1972 season lost in the pro-championship finals seven times in ten years, sometimes in the seventh game, sometimes in the last minute. I have seen all sides of this game, and as much as it hurts I'll try to suggest how the player should handle not only victory but also defeat.

In 1972, the Lakers reached the NBA playoff finals for the eighth time in my twelve seasons as a pro and we finally won, beating New York and capturing the championship which had eluded me all those years. I'm not sure if it completely made up for all those disappointments which preceded it, but it was a tremendous thrill, the greatest of my career.

Win or lose—but, of course, winning most of all—it is a great game to play. I am proud that I have generally been on winning teams if not title teams and a player

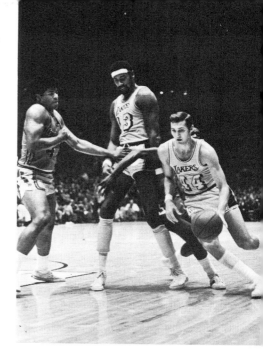

As Wilt Chamberlain blocks out my guard, I "scissors" around only to find the great Wes Unseld moving over to defense me. It sometimes seems there is not a soft spot in all of pro ball. The players who reach this level have gone as far as you can go in this game. (Photography, Inc.)

who has had the opportunity to play with the best. I have had times when I whooped with joy and times when I wept with disappointment.

Aside from my family, basketball has been the biggest and best thing in my life. When I stop playing I will miss it enormously. And I envy enormously most of you reading this book who are just beginning to play the game or will be playing it for a long while. I hope the things I have to say will help.

2. Dribbling

We're feeling plenty of pain as a foe gets wedged between Wilt Chamberlain and me as I turn a tight corner in dribbling around my teammate's block. Wilt was anchored for a legal block and I had the right of way, so our foe was at fault. This time. (Photography, Inc.)

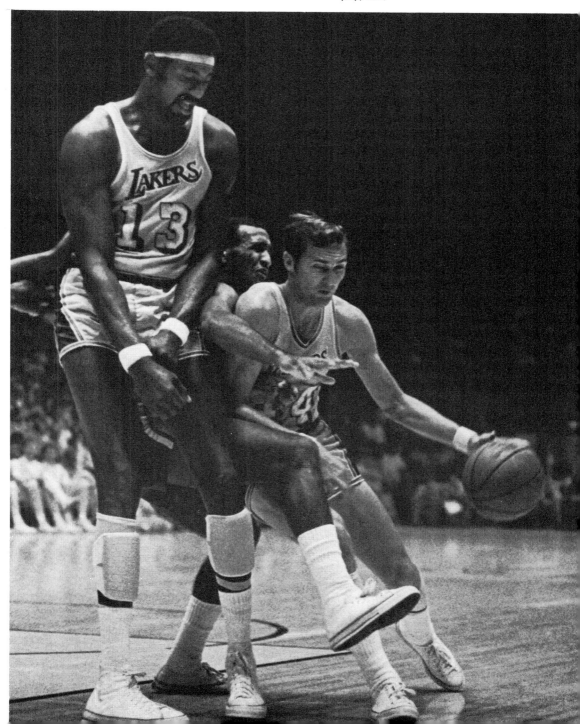

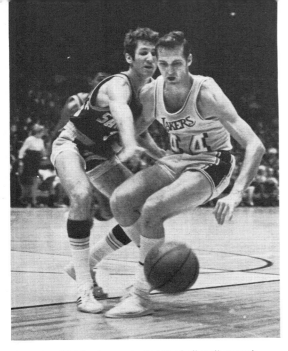

Not having protected the ball well enough on my dribble, it is batted away by a rival. (Photography, Inc.)

Teaching my son David, I stress that he bend over the ball with his knees flexed comfortably, have his hand flat to the floor with fingers spread and push it down with a relaxed rhythm. He has dropped his left hand, however, when it should be up for protection and balance. Still, he is a promising dribbler. (Photography, Inc.)

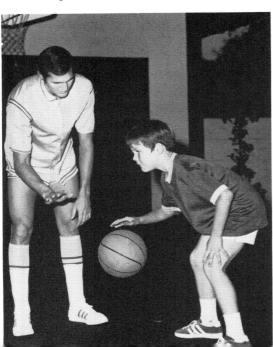

BALLHANDLING is the first art of basketball, because control of the ball is critical. You can only score when you have the ball. To score, you must move the ball. And you can move it only by dribbling or passing. The player must know how to get free to pass and to receive a pass. You protect a lead by dribbling or passing the ball.

Players with larger hands, longer fingers, and a natural sense of rhythm and timing have an advantage as dribblers, but dribbling is a skill that can with practice be learned and mastered by all. The player can practice alone before exposing himself to defensive pressure.

I'm sorry to admit that dribbling has long been the weakest part of my game. I didn't control the ball as well as I should have and often had it stolen; I also lost control of it or kicked it out of bounds a lot. Thus I have worked on dribbling more than on other parts of my game and have improved a lot. Oddly enough, I think I learned and improved the most while teaching at basketball summer camps. The act of teaching, of concentrating on it, helped. And I'd have two or three or four boys surround me and try to take the ball away from me while I dribbled, which pushed me to improve.

You dribble primarily with your fingers and wrist, although elbow-action and arm-action also enter into it. Your knees should be relaxed and bent, your body bent slightly forward from the waist, your head held erect. You bounce the ball about a foot away from your body and to the same side as the hand you are using. Your fingers are spread slightly over the top portion of the ball.

You do not slap at the ball, but you push it down with wrist-snap and lesser elbow-snap. You do not reach for it, but let it return to your hand. Receiving it, your wrist flexes back and your arm bends back to cushion it. You almost catch it, but you do not. It is a fine line. Assuming you are capable of catching it in one hand, if you do grasp it for even a split-second, you will be called for "palming the ball," which is a violation that will cost you possession of the ball. Also, you cannot turn your hand over.

Most players will tell you that you touch the ball only with your fingers and that you should never permit your palm to come in contact with the ball. I believe that while your fingers do most of the work, you cushion it and control it best by placing the pads of your hand as well as your fingers on the ball. When I am dribbling, my fingers are more forward on the ball because at all times the center of the contact made with the ball must be directly on top of it. Experiment to find what is most comfortable for you.

Begin by dribbling slowly. Do not push the ball down too hard. Push it with only enough force to bring it back to your hand solidly. Gradually increase the force of your push and the speed of your dribble until you reach the most forceful and fastest dribble you can control. Strive to increase your limits in practice, but never dribble beyond the degree of control you have mastered in games. Practice dribbling as slowly as possible, too. Once you have mastered varying speeds, you can change tempos while dribbling to keep the defenders off balance.

You are not allowed to touch the ball with both hands at the same time while dribbling, but you can and should change hands while dribbling. The player must practice with both hands. The right-hander must learn to dribble as well with his left hand as with his right hand. This is not easy and it does not come naturally, but it will come with practice. And it is critical. Here basketball differs from most sports. The switch-hitter has an advantage in baseball, but most need only bat from one side. You throw the ball with only one hand in baseball or football. But in basketball a player simply must be able to dribble or make certain passes or certain shots with either hand, otherwise his movements will be ex-

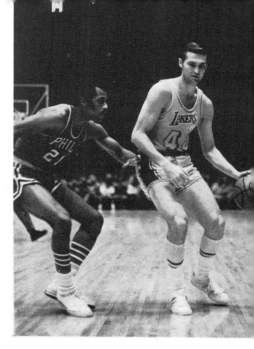

Here I have my body turned to protect the ball from Archie Clark. I am dribbling with the hand farthest from him, my left, and the pads of my hand are flush on the ball, which, in contrast to the advice of many, I recommend. I am dribbling slowly here, maneuvering for position. (Photography, Inc.)

Dribbling with his left hand, Jeff Mullins seeks to move around me. (Photography, Inc.)

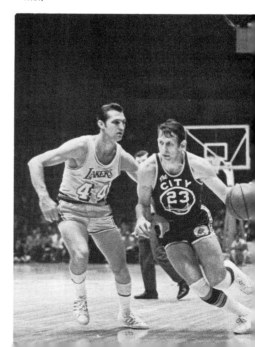

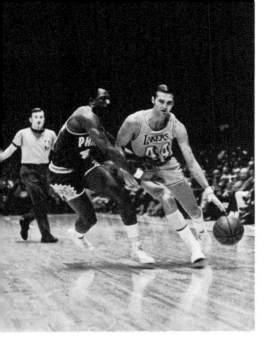

I look a bit shifty-eyed here, but as I turn a corner on Stan McKenzie, the ball low and off my left hand, I sneak a look to see what is happening under the basket and where the defenders are moving. I am not watching the ball. (Photography, Inc.)

Chased by Earl Monroe, I have broken into the open, am moving fast, and thus am dribbling high. (Photography, Inc.)

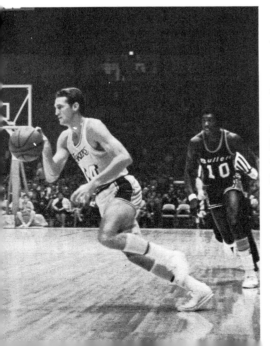

tremely limited, which gives a great edge to the defenders.

Unlike baseball, keep your eyes off the ball. You may be more comfortable during the learning process observing your dribbling action, but as soon as possible shift your gaze to a point beyond your dribble, then to a higher point on the sidelines, then to various points around the court. Work on it until you can control the ball completely and even change hands on your dribble without looking at the ball. You must keep your head and your eyes up or you will not be able to see what your defender is doing or how the play is developing in front of you.

Begin by dribbling at a height that feels most comfortable to you, which probably will be somewhere around waist-level. Then practice dribbling as high and as low as you comfortably can with control. Generally, the lower you dribble, the better. The closer a defender is to you, the lower you want to dribble. You are then exposing the ball less, reducing the chance of a steal.

However, the lower you dribble, the slower you move. Except for a pure control situation when you are simply trying to kill time, the object of dribbling is to move the ball into an attacking and passing position. The faster you move, the higher you will have to dribble. The higher you dribble, the more forcefully you will have to push the ball, the faster the tempo will become, and the less control you will have. And the higher you dribble, the more erect your posture will become. But never dribble so high that you are standing up straight and your knees are locked, because then you are most vulnerable to a steal and have the least mobility.

The lower the dribble the greater the control of the dribble, thus shorter players are usually the better dribblers. They are closer to the court to begin with. However, there is absolutely no reason why taller players, bending and flexing, cannot learn to control the ball with effective dribbling. Most, figuring they will not be the ones to bring the ball upcourt, simply do not bother to practice as much as the little guards. However, it can be a tremendous weapon for tall men. It can enable them to move around the court and into the best places from which to shoot and pass with a mobility a tall defender cannot contain. Although 7-1, Kareem Abdul-Jabbar is a brilliant dribbler, and it is one of his most surprising and effective weapons. He is not awkward moving the ball. He can escape trapping defensive pressure by dribbling. Twice he went the length of the court for layups in the 1972 playoffs against us.

The good dribbler can dribble almost as fast as he can run without the ball. He will be taking long strides. As you switch from a standing dribble to a moving dribble, you push the ball at a forward angle instead of straight down so it "leads" you. The faster you move, the greater the angle of push. If the ball is not pushed far enough in front of you, you will run into it, it will bounce off your knee, or you will kick it. However, it never should be pushed so far in front that you have to reach uncomfortably for it.

Control remains the critical factor. Practice will teach you how fast you can move while dribbling and how far you can and must push the ball in front to maintain complete control. Practice to stretch your limits, but, again, never reach for limits beyond your ability. Knowing your limitations is as important to your success as knowing your abilities.

When dribbling with the right hand, your weight may be shifted slightly to the left, and vice-versa. The point here is to maintain body control, to avoid leaning to one side or the other except when changing directions.

To change your dribble from one hand to the other, simply angle the ball from the dribbling hand toward the other while bringing the other toward the ball, slightly angled to receive it before flattening your hand out to

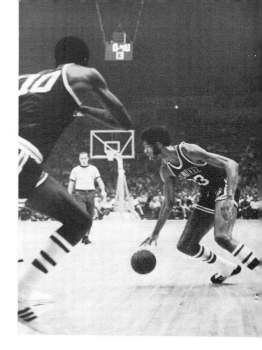

A brilliant dribbler for a big man, note how 7-footer Jabbar is flexed, bending over the ball, staying low and keeping it low to control it. (Photography, Inc.)

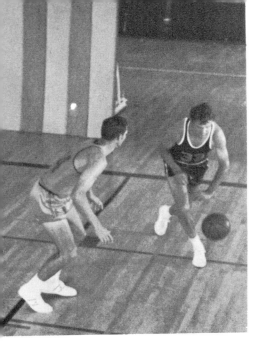

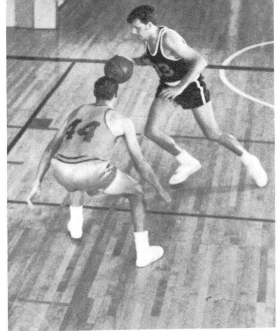

In practice, former teammate Rod Hundley going to his left, then turning to his right, switches the ball from his left hand to his right as he executes the cut on me. (William Eastabrook for Sunkist Growers)

resume the up-and-down motion. "Palming" is very much a risk here, so the angle of the receiving hand can be only slight. If you are changing hands while advancing, the ball must also be angled forward, of course.

The best way to change directions while dribbling is also to change hands. If you wish to cut to the left while dribbling with your right hand, you angle the ball to your left when your right foot strikes the ground and you push off to the left with it. Your weight is thus shifted to the left. You "receive" the ball with your left hand while your right foot crosses over to the left. The sharper the cut the more effective, but it is difficult to control the ball while cutting, so never exceed your limitations.

Begin by practicing gradual turns of direction, then, little by little, increase the sharpness of your shift. This is an invaluable weapon for bringing the ball upcourt under defensive pressure.

The dribbler has the advantage over the defender, since the dribbler knows where he is going. The dribbler should not betray his direction by looking in that direction or shifting his weight or the angle of his body, as

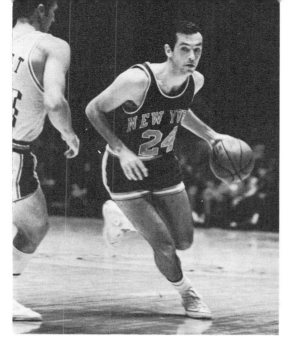

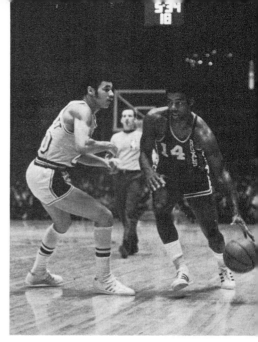

many defenders will detect it. A player can use those movements as fakes, sometimes going in that direction, sometimes not.

Another way of reversing directions on the dribble is the pivot. From a right-handed dribble the ball is angled slightly to the left and sharply inside toward the body as your right foot strikes the court and you push off to the left and shift your weight to the left, pulling your left shoulder and left side back and around toward your right. As your left hand receives the ball it is pushed back down and angled still farther to the left as you complete your swing around.

Once your back is to the defender you continue dribbling and back in to the basket or whatever position you wish to occupy. However, if the defender has taken a firm stand you cannot simply back into him and push him aside. I am not greatly in favor of backing in, because the play is behind you and you cannot see what is developing, so I seldom do it. But it is an effective weapon, especially for players with a good hook-shot or turnaround jump-shot, and for big, strong players who want to muscle in close to the basket.

Three outstanding ballhandlers—Bill Bradley (upper left) who carried Princeton to its greatest heights; Oscar Robertson (upper right) who took the University of Cincinnati to the top; and Guy Rodgers (below) who starred in his undergraduate days for Temple and could do tricks with the ball. (Photography, Inc.)

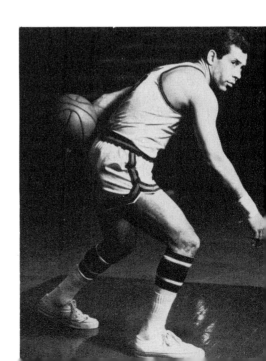

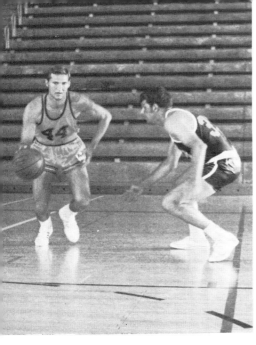

Some players shift direction sharply and effectively with a behind-the-back dribble. The ball is dribbled to the side of the body, which is permitted to move ahead of the ball, and, with a sharply cocked wrist, the ball is angled forward and to the side to the opposite hand and the dribble is resumed. This is a very difficult maneuver that takes a great deal of practice to perfect. It is usually a showboating tactic and thus of little real value. I have done it maybe a dozen times in my career, but some use it fairly often. Bob Cousy did it frequently and, while it was showy, it was an effective weapon in his hands, confusing defenders enormously.

Here is a graphic photo study of a reverse dribble that frees me for a shot. I am driving on Hundley hard to my right, I come to a sharp stop while continuing to dribble, reverse my weight, pivot around, shifting the ball from one hand to the other, and, before Rod can get back to stop me, I have come to a quick stop and gone straight up for a jump-shot. Rod was quick, but my knowing what I was going to do gave me the half-step I needed. (William Eastabrook for Sunkist Growers)

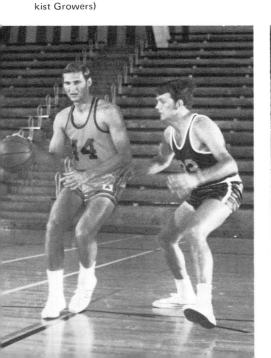

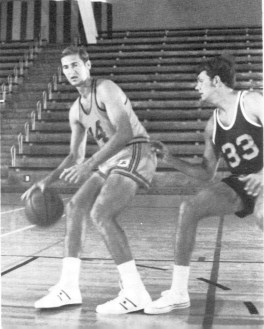

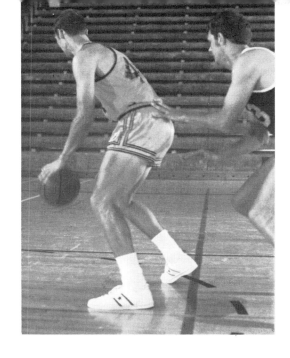
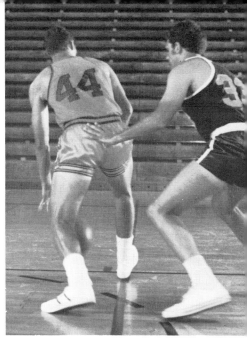
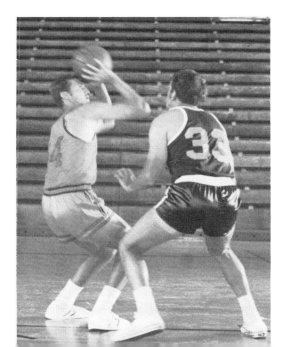
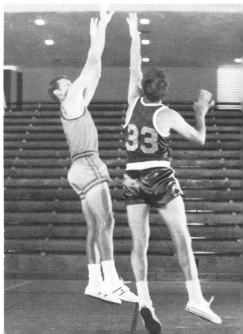

Dribbling between your legs, right to left or left to right, is a bit less difficult and, although a showboating trick, it is sometimes helpful as a deceptive maneuver.

Always dribble with the hand farthest from the defender, using your body as a shield. If he is going to lunge to steal the ball, make him go the farthest possible distance to reach it. As you learn to dribble, don't drop the opposite hand so it is dangling uselessly at your side. Keep it up and out where it can help you maintain your balance, shift your body weight and direction, and keep your defender at a greater distance. You can't use it as a club to hammer him away, but if it is up and to the side or in front of you it is an obstacle that he cannot hammer away, either.

Use changes of pace and direction of your body and dribble to keep the defender off balance. Change hands and execute cuts to keep him the greatest distance from the ball. Watch his shoulders and feet to see if he is leaning to one side or the other, then go in the opposite direction. If you see that he has shifted his weight to the heels of his feet and is leaning backward, you have him set up for a shift of direction. If you see that he has shifted his weight to the balls of his feet and is leaning forward, you have him set up for an acceleration "against the grain," which will carry you right past him. If you see his hands are up, held high, you will know he is most vulnerable to a dribble.

Under pressure, resist the tendency to turn around and back into the defender. It sometimes seems the safest thing to do, but it takes away your mobility, your ability to strike fast to one side or the other, and your ability to see the play developing.

Always practice dribbling right or left so you can go to either side with equal dexterity and so your defender cannot overplay you to one side or the other. When I first came up I always dribbled to my right. Pros soon recognized this and overplayed me to the right and hampered me enormously. I still dribble more to the right than to the left, because I have never been comfortable dribbling to my left, which is a failing. But I have practiced dribbling to my left and now defenders can no longer count on me going only to my right and cannot overplay me to any great degree.

Going to your right, dribble with your right hand— and vice-versa. No matter which way you go, look both ways. The greater a player's peripheral vision, the greater his chance of seeing openings. Some players have better peripheral vision than others. Some can look straight ahead, yet at the same time see on both sides. This is a great advantage for the dribbler or passer. To some extent it can be built up with concentration. And you can develop a slight movement of your head from side to side, which enables you to sweep over a wide area with your eyes and see not only what your teammates are doing, but what the defenders are doing.

If double-teamed, pass the ball or stop and look for a pass. Do not try to dribble between two defenders. And do not try to dribble too long while two defenders are pressing in on you, because they will swiftly get an angle on the ball. There simply is no way to keep the ball away from the defense when there are men angling in on you from both sides. The best way to move the ball is by passing it. Dribble it only to gain territorial advantage when there is not a good pass to make.

Never begin your dribble when you have no place to go. The natural tendency of most young players is to begin a dribble the minute they get the ball. But if they do not have a plan in mind they are wasting the weapon the dribble should be.

Resist being driven by defensive pressure into a corner from which there is no escape. Look for open areas and head for them. If you are being forced toward a corner, start toward it, then swiftly reverse toward an opening. If you dribble before you have a place to go to you will have to stop and will be stuck.

Never move faster than you have to. If you are be-

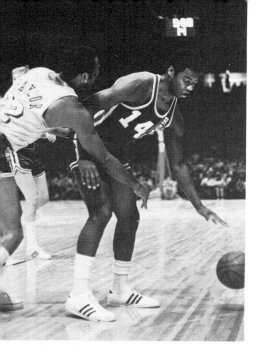

Talking of being relaxed, no one makes it
look easier than Oscar Robertson, the master all-around ballhandler, here dribbling
calmly, taking his time against the reaching
defense of Elgin Baylor. (Photography, Inc.)

hind and time is running out, obviously you have to get
the ball into an attacking position as soon as possible.
But save your speed for accelerations and shifts of speed
that will throw your defenders off stride.

Don't shift directions needlessly. Save it for when it
will help you. Don't do anything just because it is
showy. Don't throw fakes carelessly. The more fakes
you make the more difficult it is for you to control your
body and dribble. Save your fakes. Don't give anything
away. Use only what you need when you need it. Don't
waste motion and energy. Save your weapons and risk
no moves that could cost you control of the ball.

Get to know your defenders. Get to know the ones
who gamble the most, who make the same mistakes, who
are most prone to taking fakes. And get to know the
ones who have the most intelligence and greatest determination, those with the longest arms, quickest hands,
and fastest reflexes. Take more liberties with the gam-
blers and the careless defenders.

There have been many great dribblers in pro basketball, and more come along all the time. I suppose Bob
Cousy, the former Boston star, was as good as any. He
was flashy, but his flashiness was built on a base of
sound fundamentals. Oscar Robertson is a great dribbler.
His entire game stresses economy of motion. He is more
concerned with getting the job done than looking good
doing it. But he is so graceful that he can't help but look
good. He simply doesn't waste motion. Len Wilkens has
been another sound dribbler.

When you think of dribblers you often think of
Marquis Haynes, the former Harlem Globetrotter and
touring court clown. The Globetrotters and teams like
them always have a player like Haynes who dribbles
behind his back, through his legs, on his knees, even
sitting down, and at some time or another in their games
bedevils a swarm of confused foes. Well, this is great fun

and obviously a fellow has to have mastered the art to perform in this way, but most of what they do has little practical purpose in games, except possibly to stall to protect a lead at the end of high school and college games. And, except for the possibility of such a dribbler drawing fouls, a passing game is preferable for stalling situations, since it is less risky.

Anyway, most top pro dribblers could dribble this way if they wished. Calvin Murphy can and has given exhibitions of it. Pete Maravich has these kind of dribbling abilities. So does Walt Hazzard. Em Bryant, Walt Frazier, and Earl Monroe are super dribblers. Guy Rodgers long was one of the best.

Among big men, Elgin Baylor was and Connie Hawkins is exceptional. Elgin, at 6-5, used the dribble mainly as a means to get open for a shot, and he had such complete control over the ball that the Laker broadcaster, Chick Hearn, gave Baylor's dribble a name—the "yo-yo" dribble. Under Elgin's hand the ball seemed to be on a string. Elg was mainly a right-handed dribbler. He was not as good with his left.

Hawkins, even bigger at 6-8, is a masterful dribbler for a man his size. And Kareem Abdul-Jabbar, who is well over 7 feet tall, has made himself as good a dribbler for a center as any I've ever known. His body is flexible and he has more natural grace, agility, and speed than most men anywhere near his size. Hawkins and Jabbar are willing to bend a bit to get down over the ball, which most tall men, standing stiffly erect, do not do. Thus Hawkins can reach places under pressure most forwards cannot, and Jabbar is by far the most maneuverable of centers.

I'm not a good dribbler. Do as I say, not as I do. And watch others who are masters of the art. Each has his own way, but the essence of what they all do is similar. The player who wishes to improve can educate himself

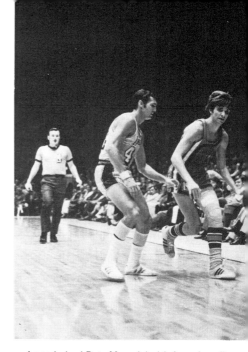

Long-haired Pete Maravich, his knee heavily bandaged, dribbles down the sidelines against my guarding. Pistol Pete, the all-time NCAA scoring champion from LSU, is one of the showiest dribblers and passers to come along. (Photography, Inc.)

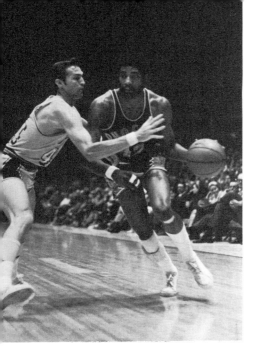

One of the big men who can really handle the ball, Connie Hawkins, bent just right and in perfect balance, cuts hard against me. I'm reaching in and shifting my feet fast to keep in range, and if I'm not careful I'll foul him. (Photography, Inc.)

sometimes not to look at a game as a whole, as a spectacle, but to break it down into its component parts, to watch certain men doing the things they do best. I don't advise anyone to simply copy a great dribbler, but there is much to be learned from all.

In moving as much as you are permitted to move with the ball without dribbling, one foot must be planted while you are permitted to swing this way and that with the other foot. Once you have established a free foot and a pivot foot, you cannot reverse them until you have dribbled or given up the ball.

When you begin your dribble your pivot foot cannot leave the floor until the ball has left your hand. If you are beginning a shot your pivot foot is permitted to leave the floor, but it cannot return to the court until the ball has left your hand or you will be guilty of an infraction.

You may take as many steps as you wish while dribbling. If when you stop your dribble one foot is in the air, the planted foot must then remain your pivot foot. You have no choice. If you stop with two feet on the court you have a choice. Clearly, this is preferable. Some players are more comfortable using the same foot as a pivot foot all the time. The same rule applies to receiving a pass, incidentally. If, for example, you must reach for a pass and catch it with one foot in the air, you are stuck with the planted foot as your pivot foot.

In dribbling, even at top speed, one of the advantages of having your legs spread comfortably, your knees bent, and your body flexed at the waist is that you will be better able to stop on both feet in balance without your forward thrust toppling you toward an extra and illegal step. Some players use a two-foot jump-stop and some a stride-stop. In the first they sort of give a little jump, landing, sort of planting themselves, with both feet as they stop. In the other they take a longer-than-usual stride and bend lower than usual in coming to a halt. Both are effective.

When you are coming to a stop off a dribble, grasp the ball in both hands, pull it in to your belly, and bend over it, elbows extended, to protect it with your body. Once you are set you can move the ball around, but it is at that moment before you are set, such as immediately after a dribble, when the player is often especially vulnerable to having it batted or taken from his hands.

Remember, the point of dribbling is to gain a territorial advantage. Almost all players can develop a rhythmic dribbling ability, but save the showmanship for the stage. More people will pay to see winners than the most colorful of losers. The gyms and playgrounds are full of *former* players who can fool around with a lot of flash.

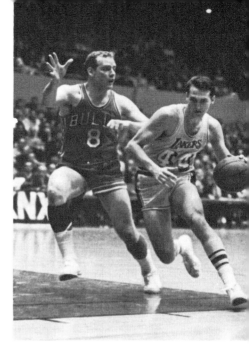

Trying to turn a corner on a rival who has a good angle on me, I grab the ball in both hands and tuck it in my belly to protect it while coming to a stop with both feet. From here I probably will have to pass off, though if I go right up for a quick jumper I may catch him anchored to the court with the momentum of his sudden stop. (Photography, Inc.)

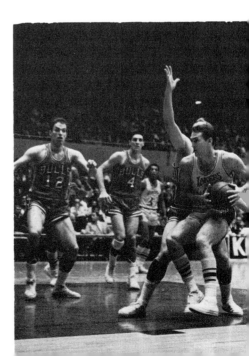

3. Passing

Here I pass back out over Bob Rule and Len Wilkens after getting trapped under the basket. (Photography, Inc.)

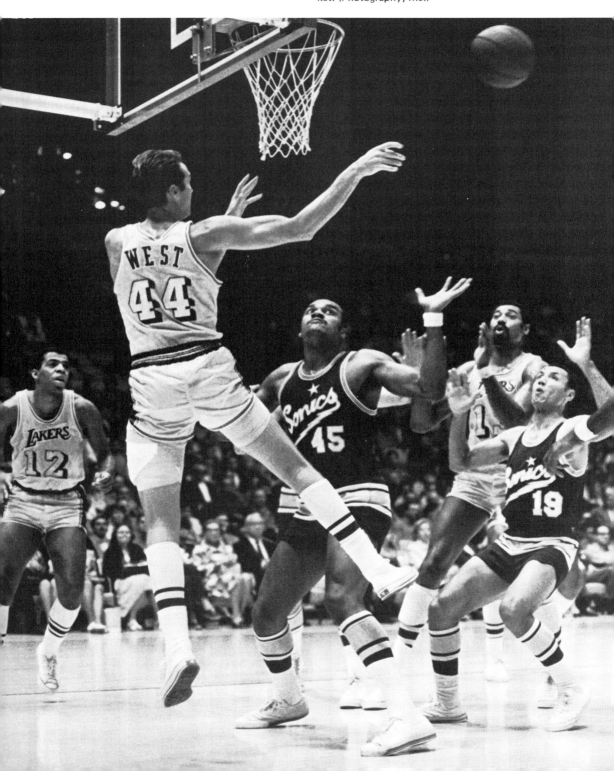

THE SECOND part of ballhandling is the passing game. If you can't get the ball to the shooters in position for their best shots, you can't score. It is perhaps the most important skill for the small player to stress, since it is expected of him, but it is also a key area in which the taller player can strengthen his overall game and his value to his team. The center needs passing and receiving skills, since many plays are run off the pivot. And the forward needs these skills, because he often operates in a congested corner.

Passing offers an enormous opportunity to the player. Sometimes it will show up in the statistics, sometimes it won't. They keep a record of assists, which are passes that lead directly to baskets, but these don't tell the whole story. A good player controls the game with his passing. This is especially true of guards, since they'll usually bring the ball upcourt and begin the offensive play. But passing is important in all positions. The center who gets his hands on the ball a great deal can help his team enormously with passes.

When the situation calls for it, pass on the run, off the dribble. Provided you do not lose your precision, the sooner you penetrate the defense the less it is likely to have set up in position. The quicker and harder you pass the less likely that the defender will anticipate it, deflect it, or steal it.

However, never make an awkward pass and never force a pass. If you do not have good control of your body coming off the dribble, do not try for the pass. Always be sure your momentum does not cause you to pass harder than you had planned. Pass only when the intended receiver is expecting it. It does no good to deceive the opposition if you deceive your teammate at the same time.

Some players are better able to handle difficult passes than are others. Some are more alert to passing possibilities. Know your teammates. Don't complain about

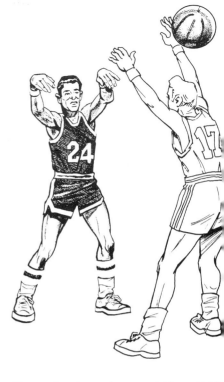

The two-hand pass, thrown quickly and high through the outspread arms of a defender.

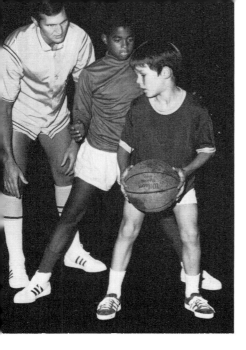

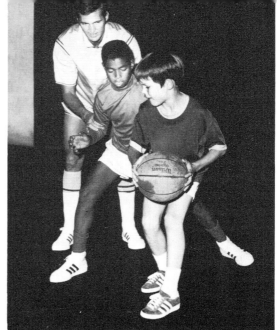

Son David is tutored in the art of pivoting off a foot, in this case his right, relieving the pressure of defender Kevin Hawkins and seeking a lane to pass through. (Photography, Inc.)

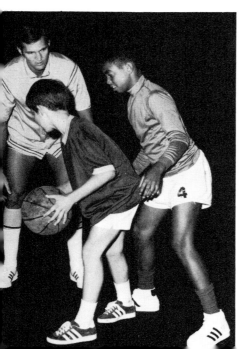

them; adjust to them. Make the passes each can handle. It is the passer who determines the pass he's going to make, when he's going to make it, and who's going to get it.

Once you stop with the ball, you can move your free foot as much as you wish as long as your pivot foot remains anchored. You may swivel on your pivot foot, but you may not slide the foot forward or raise it. As with starting and especially stopping, pivoting seems a simple maneuver that does not require much practice, but it is deceptively difficult to execute well and requires a great deal of practice.

You must protect the ball. Hold it firmly with both hands on either side of the ball and your fingers spread. Hold it in to your body with your elbows bent and angled out and your body bent over it. Give the ball maximum protection as you pivot. Always try to keep the ball at the greatest distance from your defender, if possible with your body between the ball and the defender. Pivot on the ball of your pivot foot and try to remain balanced at all times. Do not stride so far with your free foot or turn so sharply that you lose your balance.

While dribbling or pivoting, or while simply holding the ball, you can use some fakes to confuse your foe. A step or a look in one direction, a shake of the head or shoulders, will tend to fool your defender. A short, swift shake of the ball in one direction might also confuse him. Then if you quickly move yourself or the ball in another direction you will have a good chance of completing the play. However, if you always make a preliminary fake in one direction, then attempt to execute a play in another, your smarter foes will soon spot it and take advantage of it. You should mix up your moves. You should never use too many fakes. Save them for when they're needed.

I believe that too many players use too many fakes—on every level, but especially on the lower levels. The young player seems inclined to showiness. After a while the fakes are ignored and all he has done is wear himself out. This applies to shooting as well as dribbling and passing.

Elgin Baylor had a sort of nervous twitch, a quick snap of his facial features that came out on court, especially when he was younger. He could not control it, but he never let it bother him. At one time there were some who thought it indicated he could not stand up to pro pressures. I needn't point out how wrong these people were. And what Elg had was a sort of built-in fake, which foes fought to ignore.

One of the most fundamental fakes a player can use when he has the ball and before he has begun his dribble is the "rocker step." In this he simply takes a stride forward as if he were going to begin a dribble-drive in that direction, which hopefully will put his defender off balance. He then draws back as if about to shoot or pass over the defender, which tends to draw the defender in. He can then take that quick step to the defender's side and dribble-drive past him.

Speed is a player's greatest asset. I am not speaking strictly of running speed. The fastest players in full stride are not always the ones who can commence their moves with the quickest moves. I am speaking of quickness of mind, eye, hand, and foot. Some players are naturally quicker than others, but a great deal of quickness can be developed. The key thing lies in making your moves decisively without hesitation. Decide what you are going to do and then do it, right then. The quick move will upset your opponent more than any fake. In passing, as in dribbling and shooting, you have a built-in advantage, as you know what you are going to do, when you are going to do it, and where you are going to do it before the defender does.

It's a cliché, but he who hesitates is lost. If you begin to make a move you cannot complete and then hesitate, if you must stop in midmove or falter at the end of your move, you will have lost one of those little battles that make up the war that is each game. Lose too many little battles and you will lose the war. As you play, even as you practice, you will learn what you can and can't do. Again, keep trying to increase the things you can do, but in games never exceed your present limitations. Use the moves you can use quickly and effectively and you will be making the most of your own ability.

Bill Russell, who led Boston to eleven playoff titles in thirteen seasons, did it with great defending and rebounding, but also with passing. He calls it "orchestrating games." By this he means seeing that all his teammates got their best shots. This is a subtle thing. A man may be open, but he may not be in a place from which he shoots best. The secret to good passing is getting it to the right man in the right place at the right time.

If a player gets open in the right place at the right time and does not get the ball, he is going to feel frustrated. If this happens a few times, he may get upset and say to himself that the next time he gets the ball he's not going to pass it, he's going to shoot it. It would be hard

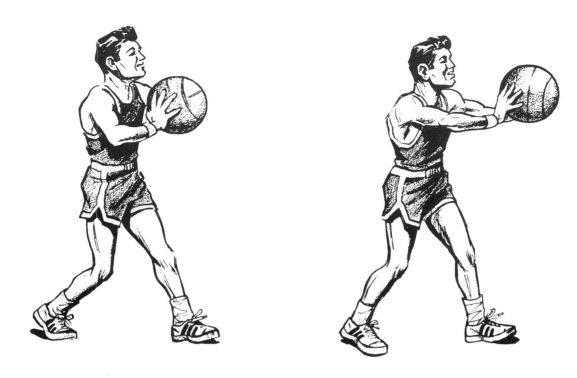

The basic two-hand chest pass.

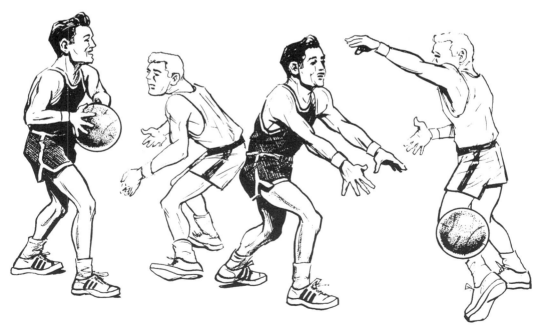

An opening to the side through which the passer throws a two-hand bounce pass.

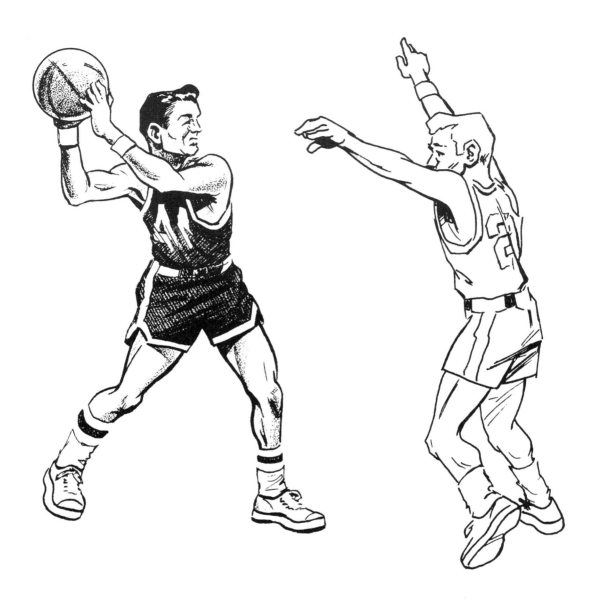

Holding the ball away in both hands, the
passer lures the defender into a move, then
throws a one-hand pass to the other side.

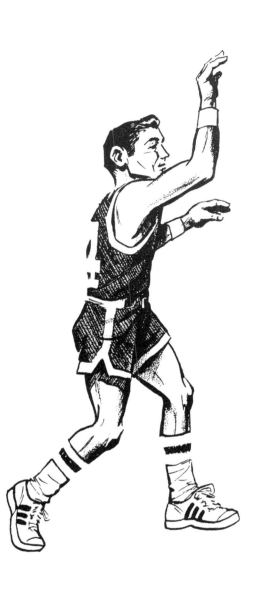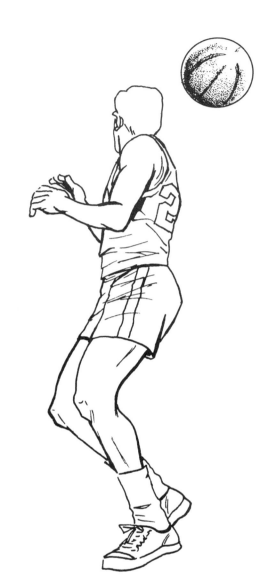

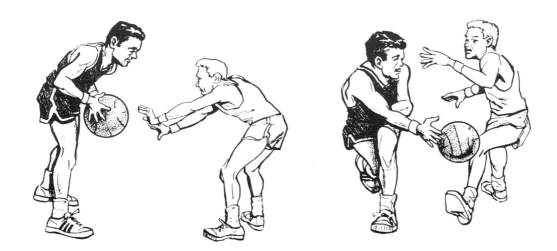

The cross-over with a one-hand bounce pass.

for him to do anything worse on a basketball court. You can't let your ego get in the way of proper play. You have to let the game situation and the defense dictate your moves. You can't make up your mind to pass or shoot before you see how the play develops. You can't pass only to friends. All teammates have to be the same to you on court. Should one of your teammates be playing selfishly, you still have to resist doing so yourself.

One of the biggest problems in playing the game on the lower levels is that cliques tend to develop and a few fellows get most of the passes and take most of the shots while their teammates are wasted. A player does have to be selective. If his best shots come up he should take them. But if an open teammate has a better shot he should get the ball. The passer has to know what passes his teammates can handle best, where their best shots are, and which are the best shooters. But he shouldn't get carried away with his own judgment. He has to see that everyone gets his share of chances.

Some players have what we call "board hands." They

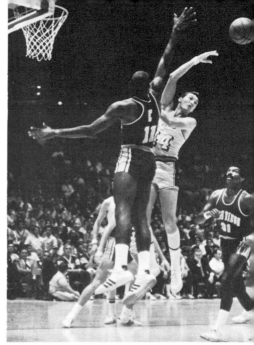

just don't catch the ball very well. Some of these may be good shooters, however, so you still have to get the ball to them. You just don't try difficult passes to them. You wait until you can make a sure pass. Actually, you wait until you can make a sure pass to any player. It's just that some players can handle a wider variety of passes and more difficult passes. If it's a pass the receiver can handle, and it's a pass you feel you should make, well, then, make it.

Never force a pass. If you have doubts you can complete a pass, hang on to the ball, even if you're under pressure. If you're tied up, you still have a chance of regaining control on the jump ball. If you throw a bad pass and lose the ball, it's gone. The player who gets the ball in good position and has mastered a wide variety of passes will find a pass he can make most of the time.

Fancy passes, such as those behind your back or through your legs, seldom have any real value. Few players can execute these effectively very often, and even if they can—what's the point? To look flashy? Occasionally, under great defensive pressure, you may be driven to such passes as your only way to get the ball to a teammate, but use such passes only if you have control of them. Never just "get rid of the ball." As part of a team you have accepted a responsibility to handle the ball and do the best possible things with it. Don't overpass. Don't just throw the ball around for the sake of doing something. Make every pass count. It's safest.

Threading the needle by slipping a surprise pass through a maze of players to a teammate can be a beautiful thing in the hands of a master, but only players with exceptional vision, imagination, timing, quickness, strength, and touch can execute such passes consistently. In watching pros, don't imitate things beyond you. Practice and use only those passes you've perfected. Anyway, more such passes seem to go astray than succeed. Even if they get through the defenders, they often seem

Passing from difficult positions, such as when stymied off a dribble or after a shot attempt, is shown in these photos. Above, from under and behind the backboard, I pass over Bob Rule and Lenny Wilkens. Wilt Chamberlain waits expectantly in the background. Below, the only escape I had from the leaping defense of Elvin Hayes was to hook a pass to a mate. Again trapped in midair, I send the ball overhand over the defense of Luke Jackson to a teammate while Jim Washington watches. (Photography, Inc.)

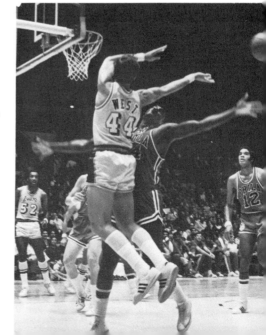

to go through the receiver, too. When a couple of players master such situations and team together smoothly, then such passes are worthwhile.

Personally, I favor short, high, hard, direct passes because these are the easiest to control and catch. Never pass carelessly. Always use the easiest pass that will work in a given situation. The closer you are to the receiver, the better your chances of reaching him with the pass and not having it deflected or intercepted. Most players prefer to catch passes chest-high, and this puts them in the best position to take a quick shot or make a quick pass, so try for this whenever possible. The harder the pass the less likely your foes can react to it in time. Of course, you don't want to throw a too-hot-to-handle pass.

A lot of guys are always running around with their hands up yelling they're open no matter where they are. If they are not in position to do something good with the ball, if they have no place to go with it, there's no point in giving it to them. No pass to this man can be a good pass. But if your style of offense calls for the ball to go into the center in the pivot position a lot, it is your job to get it to him. If he is a tall man, a looping, high pass may be best, a pass he can reach up for, perhaps even jump a little for, but never throw such a soft looper if it is simply "up for grabs." The taller the player, the less likely he is to be able to handle low or bounce passes.

Tailor your passes to the opportunity and to the target. Experience enters into this a lot. You don't learn it all at once. The more you play the game, the more you get a "feel" for the right passes.

Look for a lane to throw through. Be aware where the defenders are in relation to the pass and what chance they have of getting over to pick it off. Accordingly, the worst pass usually is the length-of-the-court pass or the cross-court pass, simply because it has to travel the longest distance through or over the greatest number of players and thus is most vulnerable to being picked off.

Bill Bradley, the former Princeton all-American and Rhodes scholar, grips the ball firmly, sights a line, and prepares to make a two-hand bounce pass from his chest past Mike Lynn on defense. (Photography, Inc.)

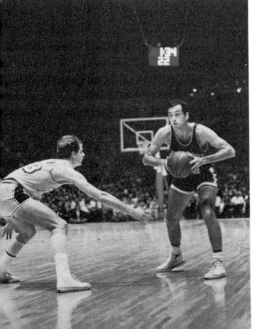

Concentration on what is developing in front of you and your peripheral vision will stand you in good stead here.

Like a good baseball pitcher, mix up your passes and learn the best kind of pass to throw in each situation. But vary the type of pass you throw and the speed of the throw as much as possible to keep potential interceptors off balance. Use fakes where necessary, but be careful not to fake out the intended receiver. Be careful not to fool your teammate with a pass he's not expecting. The only way to avoid this is to practice together. As passers and receivers get to know each other's habits they are less apt to make mistakes.

Hold the ball firmly and throw it sharply. Stride in the direction of your pass and follow through with your arm, just as a baseball pitcher or a football passer does. But since you must stride in the direction of the pass, be aware that this is a tipoff to the opposition of where you are throwing the ball. Compensate for this by making your move quickly. Try not to look directly at the receiver, but have him in your vision.

Don't throw blind passes. Pass to spots only when it has been set up in prearranged play and perfected. Learn to time lead passes. Adjust the length of the lead to the speed of your moving teammate. There is nothing more frustrating to a man breaking open for his best shot than to have the ball thrown too far in front of him or behind him. Practiced teamwork will pay off.

There are many possible passes. Each is a weapon and each can be practiced by players working out alone before they need be practiced with a partner and then eventually with a team. A player can mark spots on a wall and practice hitting these with various passes. Later, he can turn to a friend or teammate to practice hitting a moving target with various passes.

A basic pass is the two-hand chest-pass. It is used mainly for shorter passes. Be in balance with your feet spread comfortably. Flex your knees slightly and bend your body forward slightly from the waist. Spread your

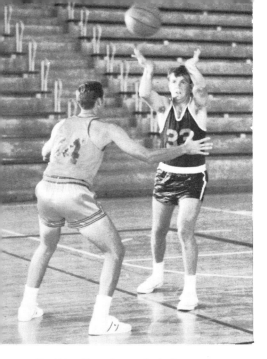

Rod Hundley releases the ball on a two-hand overhead pass over my defense in practice. The ball has been released close to him and on his straight follow-through his hands and palms turn downward. (William Eastabrook for Sunkist Growers)

I practice a two-hand bounce pass to Jim McMillian. My hands are thrust downward and my hand and fingers remain spread. The ball has been sent to the court closer to him than to me and with enough force to come up to him at waist-level. (Photography, Inc.)

fingers wide and hold the ball away from your chest with your hands to the rear of the ball, your elbows bent and angled out. The ball can be cushioned against the pads of your hands, but the fingers will do most of the work. As you pass, stride forward and snap the ball forward with a snap of the elbows and wrists. Release the ball close to your body when your motion has reached its full force, not at the full extension of your arms when your action is spent. But follow through with your hands in the direction of your pass. At the completion your palms will be spread downward. Aim for your receiver's chest. This pass usually is made sharply, with fair force, the ball spun off the fingertips.

The same pass may be executed with the ball held over or to the side of the head. The mechanics are the same. These are used when there is defensive pressure, and are not as efficient because you do not have as much control over the ball and because it is more exposed to the defenders. The overhead pass is usually used with a slight loop to get the ball to a tall pivot.

The two-handed bounce-pass is executed similarly except that the arms and hands are thrust down. The ball is bounced closer to the receiver than to the passer, since in striking the court it will lose some of its momentum. The ball should be thrust into the court hard

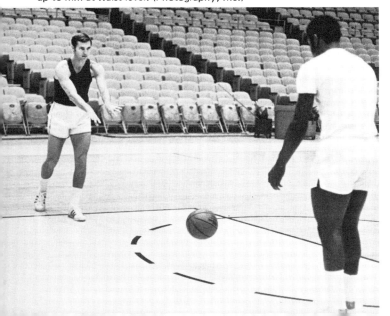

enough to reach the receiver at least waist-high, unless he
is deliberately bending over to receive such a pass low.
No such pass should be made if the ball must bounce
more than once to reach the receiver, and since the pass
cannot be as hard as a direct pass, it should not be a long
one.

Since the defenders usually have their hands high, the
low bounce-pass is often a good one. A defender can
kick the ball, but since this is illegal, possession would
revert to you. Possibly, this type of pass is not used
enough.

The over-the-shoulder pass and the bounce-pass can
be executed successfully with one hand, too, though
obviously you do not have as much control of the ball.
The younger and smaller you are the more advisable it is
to use two hands and not stretch your strength limitations beyond reason.

One-hand passing has advantages, however, in that

Under the basket, Wilt Chamberlain holds
the ball high with two hands as he prepares
to pass off to me, open at the left. Willie
McCarter is open in the center but not looking for the ball. Mel Counts, defended by
Paul Silas, is beginning to move toward the
middle to free himself. (Photography, Inc.)

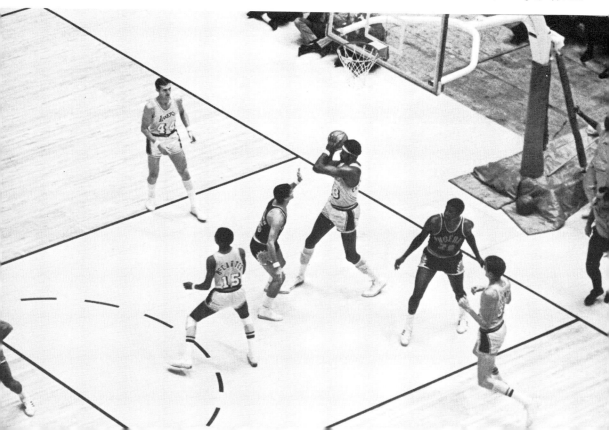

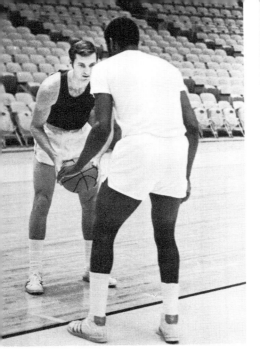

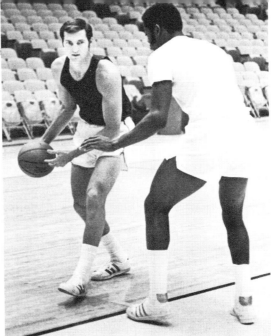

Guarded by Jim McMillian in practice, I cross over to my right and reach around him to pass off. (Photography, Inc.)

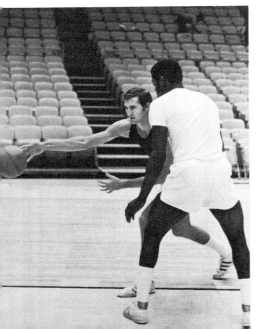

usually the pass is thrown quicker and faster. It is faster only because we are more used to throwing all kinds of balls with one hand and have a more natural motion developed for it. The one-hand bounce pass is especially effective when thrown to an open player cutting toward the basket for a layup, provided the ball is bounced high enough for him to receive it comfortably high and in full stride.

There are two types of one-handed passes that cannot be executed as effectively with two hands. One is the cross-over or reach-around pass. Under tight defensive pressure in which another kind of pass would be difficult to execute, the passer can often get the ball to a teammate by pivoting sharply and taking a long stride to one side and reaching around the defender to hook the ball back to his teammate on the opposite side.

The other is the so-called baseball pass, which really comes closer to being football's forward pass. This is used mainly for long passes, such as to launch a fast-break. A rebounder will often use it the instant he comes down with the ball as his teammates tear up the court to catch the opposition with its defenses down. Spread your feet for balance, bring the ball up to ear-level with both hands for control, draw the ball about a foot behind your head with one hand—with that hand spread behind and slightly under the ball—and, as you stride forward, snap the ball toward the intended receiver, leading him, with a full extension of your arm and hand. At the follow-through, the arm and palm of your hand are parallel to the court. Never try to throw the ball farther than you can with reasonable accuracy. Some men have mastered this pass, but many underthrow the ball into an interceptor's hands or overthrow it out-of-bounds.

There are other passes the player can make. A two-hand or one-hand underhand shovel-pass, for example, and a behind-the-back or between-the-legs pass when closely covered. There are situations in which such extreme tactics may be called for. But these are rare, and such passes should be used rarely.

Any kind of pass that gets the ball to the man you want to reach at the time and at the place you want him to get it is a great pass. The player can be flexible and work beyond the basic passes with some that he can make work. But unless you can make these passes work nine out of ten times, forget them until you can.

It is not easy to make all passes consistently. It takes practice and experience. From high up in the stands, open players and openings for passes can often be seen clearly which cannot be seen on the court, where the player is constantly screened off by a shifting maze of players. The smaller the player the less apt he is to be able to see over the heads of his foes and the more surrounded he will feel. Yet most of the best passers in basketball history have been small men, because it is more their job—they are the playmakers.

I'm a good passer. Earlier I admitted I was far from a good dribbler. I'm trying to be honest about the things I do well and the things I do not do well. I led the Lakers

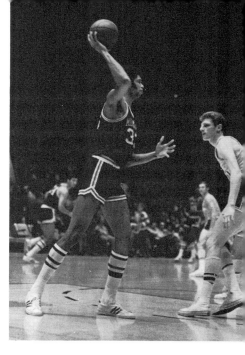

The baseball pass, which really comes closer to being a football pass and is a major way players launch fast-breaks, is illustrated here by Lew Alcindor, left, in game action against Mel Counts. (Photography, Inc.)

Rod Hundley, who is given to inventive passes, crosses over, reaches around me, and tries a two-hand pass. (William Eastabrook for Sunkist Growers)

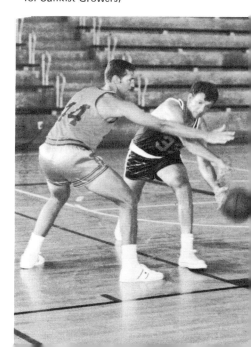

in assists eight times. In the 1971-72 season I set a team record with 747 assists and led the NBA with an average of 9.5 assists per game. However, the NBA records are held by Guy Rodgers with 908 assists in a season and Oscar Robertson with an average of 11.5 assists. Robertson holds the lifetime record with more than 8,000 assists. I'm fifth. Cousy led the NBA in assists eight times. Oscar has led six times. Cousy and Rodgers hold the record with 28 assists in a single game. I rank fourth with 23 in one game.

Bob Cousy is generally regarded as the best passer in basketball history. He was very flashy, but extremely efficient, too. He was going out as I was coming in. I think Guy Rodgers has been one of the best all-around ballhandlers, dribblers, and passers of my time. Oscar has been the best. He almost never makes a bad pass or has the ball stolen from him. He's not flashy, but he always gets the ball to the man who should get it. He orchestrated Milwaukee's march to the 1971 NBA title masterfully and probably was as responsible for their playoff success as was Kareem Abdul-Jabbar, which is saying a lot.

K. C. Jones was a fine, sure passer. Lenny Wilkens has been consistently sharp at passing. Dave Bing is very good, so is Walt Frazier. Walt Hazzard and Earl Monroe are fine, but flashy passers. Hazzard tries more difficult passes than most, can make more than most, but also misses more than most. When he was with the Lakers he made a lot of startling passes receivers weren't expecting or couldn't handle. Since then, he has, through experience, become a bit more conservative. When he teamed one season with Pete Maravich, the ball was sometimes flipped around in Globetrotter fashion. Maravich has passing skills, but he must learn not to try the ones he can't complete.

John Havlicek, who plays both forward and guard, is one of the better-passing "big men." Another was Bay-

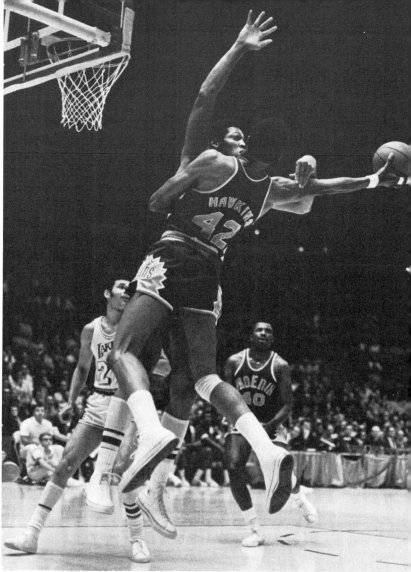

lor, who led the Lakers in assists four times. Elg had such magnificent hands and such superb control of the ball, he was a gifted passer and playmaker. He could have had many more assists if he had not shot as much, but shooting was his main job.

Connie Hawkins is another big forward who can execute stunning passes, though he sometimes tries a few too many.

An agile big man with remarkable control of his body in midair, Connie Hawkins reaches around an extremely aggressive defender to make a one-handed pass. (Photography, Inc.)

Among centers, Bill Russell was the outstanding example of a playmaking pivot who always got the ball to
the right man in the right place at the right time. Wilt
Chamberlain has been playing this position in this way a
lot in recent years and holds the NBA record for centers
with 702 assists in a single season. Kareem Abdul-Jabbar
has talent as a passer. He thinks in terms of getting the
ball to the man who should have it. He is unselfish, so he
is effective in some ways that don't show in the head-
lines.

Before concluding this chapter on ballhandling, something should be added about pass-receivers. Sometimes
too much is said about the fellows who can or can't
make good passes and not enough about the fellows who
can or can't receive them. It is an often-overlooked but
critical part of a player's talents, and this is a two-way
street. Although the passer has the major responsibility
for the success or failure of his passes, there is no doubt
but that he is often helped or hindered by the ability of
his receivers.

It is sometimes said that the truest test of a player is
his ability to move without the ball. To some extent this
is true. There are ten men on a court at any given time
and no matter how much any one player dominates a
game, he is still going to handle the ball only a limited
part of the time. The rest of the time he must be doing
something else. On offense, this consists of setting
screens, which we'll discuss in the shooting section, and
getting loose for a pass. Gail Goodrich is a master of
playing without the ball, of getting into the best position
to take a pass and make a shot. Jim McMillian is very
good, too.

The player without the ball or the player who has just
passed the ball, should break into the areas designated
for him without intruding on another player's territory.
The forwards normally work out of the corners, the
center in the middle, the guards out of the backcourt.

The receiver should look to get open in the places where he has his best shots or from which he can make the best passes. He has to look to help out his teammate with the ball, to take it from the teammate when the latter is threatened by defensive pressure. He must keep moving. He can shout for the ball when he is where he wants to be and open just as the passer can shout at the player to whom he is going to throw the ball. But both should be aware that this gives information to the enemy and requires crisp execution to overcome. The receiver should never shout selfishly while he is covered or in a useless place. This may seem obvious, but many are guilty of it.

The receiver should be aware of the types of passes his various teammates are apt to throw, how they throw them, and which ones they usually throw him. The receiver should keep his hands open and relaxed, his fingers spread, and be ready to take a pass even at what may seem to be an unexpected time. If the passer can get the ball to him, it should not be unexpected. If it is possible, it must be considered probable. The worst that will happen is that you won't be thrown the ball.

When you are thrown the ball, reach for it whenever possible and catch it in both hands. Keep your hands relaxed, but open, with your fingers slightly spread, and let your hands and elbows "give" to cushion the impact. Play the ball, don't let it play you. Whenever possible, bring the ball in to your body to protect it before making a move with it. It is on an exchange of the ball that it is most open to interception or deflection. Never make a move with it before you have it secured in your hands. Never anticipate the catch. Never consider it complete until it really is complete.

When you receive the ball on the move, such as when you are cutting for the basket, obviously you cannot step into the ball. Sometimes you may have to make the initial reception with one hand. However, always bring up the other hand to assist in securing the ball as soon as

Catching a high pass, I reach up with both hands, cushion the impact, and prepare to bring the ball down. That's Dick Garrett cutting behind me. (Photography, Inc.)

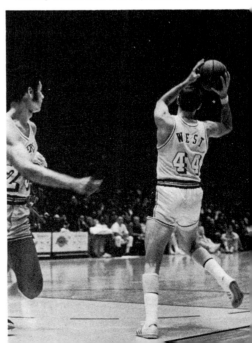

possible. Sometimes you may have to make a swift move with it, such as for a layup. In any event, you must still secure the ball before you go up with it. Frequently the ball will be muffed in this situation because the receiver must make a move before he has control of the ball. In any event, if you get the ball on the move you must shoot it or pass it or begin your dribble before you take your second step, so you must combine a fast move with precision.

Generally, you will angle your palm and fingers slightly up for high passes and slightly down for low passes, and you should always hold your hands close enough together so that a hard pass will not rip through. If your hands are not facing the ball the chances of it ripping through are greatly increased. If they are not spread, the chances of jamming your fingers or muffing the pass are increased. This is a simple enough fundamental, but it is important to build good habits here.

Know where the ball is at all times. Always expect a pass. The passer will appreciate it. It takes teamwork to have a good ballhandling club, to have a potent passing game. It takes teamwork to win.

4. Shooting

Surrounded by San Francisco Warriors, I go up two-handed for a one-hand underhand shot. (Photography, Inc.)

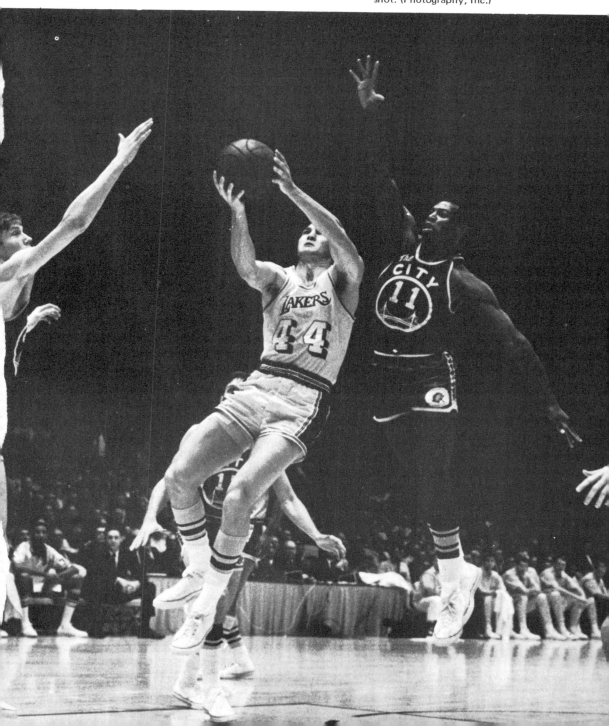

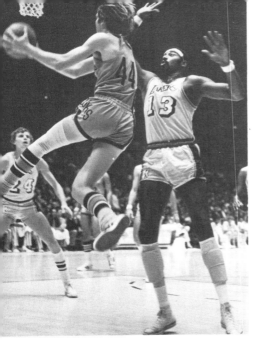

Pistol Pete Maravich, the super-scorer who has been known to force a shot or two, drives around Wilt and attempts a two-hand underhand shot from behind and beneath the basket. Keith Erickson looks on, left. (Photography, Inc.)

THE OBJECT of the game of basketball is to put a ball through a basket. It's not as easy as it sounds. The basket is hung 10 feet high on a backboard and is 18 inches in diameter; the ball is 9 inches in diameter. Many years ago the ball was worked carefully for the best shots, which usually were either two-hand set-shots from outside or layups inside. Teams scored an average of 20 to 30 points a game.

Twenty-five years ago there were pro playoff games with scores like 69-53 and 56-51. There was only one shooter in the entire NBA who hit more than 36 percent of his shots from the field. Joe Fulks, the first great scorer of pro basketball, shot 25 to 30 percent from the field. Championship college games went 43-40 and 46-45, and championship high school games 36-33 and 37-35.

Going back a bit further, when John Wooden—who at UCLA has coached more NCAA championship teams than any man ever—was in high school, his team lost the Indiana championship game, 13-12. In his time he has had to adjust to fantastic changes in the game.

The development of the fast-break with emphasis on swift dribbling, running, and ballhandling, and, more than anything else, the development of the one-hand jump-shot, have revolutionized the game to the point where high school teams average 60 to 70 points a game, college clubs 70 to 80 points, and the pro team that scores less than 100 points in a game is figured to have had an off-night.

Almost every major city in the country has high school players who average 30 points a game. This remains a fancy-enough figure for pros contesting for the scoring championship every year. I won the NBA scoring title in 1970 with an average of 31.2 points per game. However, it's hard to say what may happen in the future. Pete Maravich recently averaged more than 44 points a game for his entire three-year college career and

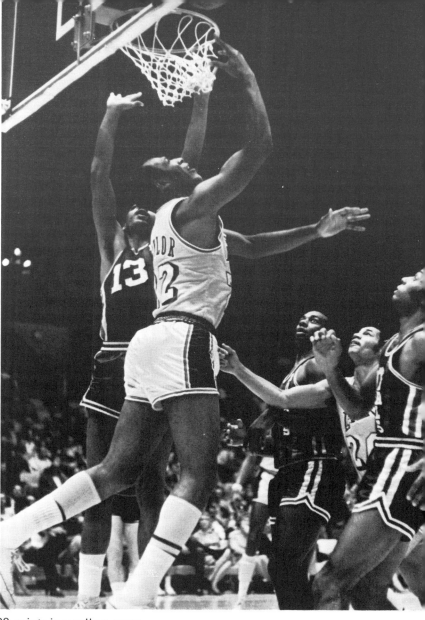

once Frank Selvy scored 100 points in a college game. Wilt Chamberlain averaged more than 50 points a game one pro season and scored 100 points in a single pro contest. Elgin Baylor holds the record for forwards with 73 points in one game.

Elgin Baylor reaches up to spin one in from behind. Oscar Robertson watches wide-eyed in the middle. (Photography, Inc.)

The emphasis on speed has not reduced shooting efficiency. On all levels the good players now hit on 40 to 50 percent of their field-shots. Wilt Chamberlain holds the one-season record in the NBA with a .683 percentage. At one time he scored 35 consecutive field-goals without a miss. Of course, the big centers, who are usually the league-leaders in percentage, take most of their shots in close. But there are many good forwards and guards, such as Lou Hudson, Jerry Lucas and Oscar Robertson who hit far over .500 every season. Dave Debusschere and Bill Bradley are great shooters.

Chamberlain is the all-time pro scoring champion with close to 30,000 points. I'm in there with Oscar, Elgin, Bob Pettit, and Hal Greer above the 20,000-point mark. It was one of the few real goals I set for myself in basketball, and when it was reached during my tenth season as a pro in 1971, I felt an enormous sense of accomplishment. I have a career shooting percentage above 47 percent and have led my Lakers in accuracy four times and scoring six times.

There is a tendency for the old-timers to tell tall-tales about the super-shooters of the past. They talk about Bob Davies and Max Zaslofsky and others who shot two-hand set-shots in the 1940's as being superior to the one-hand scat-shooting of today's players. Well, Davies usually shot 35, 36, 37 percent and Zaslofsky 31, 32, 33 percent. Bill Sharman, regarded as the peerless pro shooter of the 1950's, shot 41, 42, 43 percent. He was the best of his time. But today's outside shooters are far superior. A Lou Hudson one-hands his way to an average between 45 and 55 percent every season. I have averaged about 47 percent for my pro career. Oscar Robertson is around 50 percent every season.

I hold the NBA records for guards, with 63 points scored in one regular-season game and 53 in one playoff game. Games like this occur when you get hot, when you have a couple of streaks of eight or nine shots in a row that go in, when other players on your team are

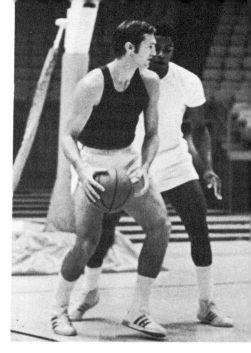

shooting so poorly that you, with the "hot hand," are inclined to shoot more than normal, when hustle brings you a few loose balls and follow-ups that result in baskets, when you get fouled enough to get 10 or 15 from the free-throw line—when the ball bounces right for you all night.

Actually, the more I play the more I consider consistency the single most important factor in evaluating a player's performance. Those big nights are fun, but over the long run I'd rather have a long string of good performances game after game than a great game one night and a poor game the next. This covers all parts of my game.

As for scoring, well, it's impossible to stop a good scorer. I really believe this. He knows what he's going to do, the defender doesn't. The only thing that can stop a good scorer is the scorer himself. Maybe he's hurting or tired or has some personal problem he permits to pester him. And some nights, for no clear reason, you just don't have the touch. When I've had a bad night and they say later that so-and-so did a great defensive job to me, I don't say anything, but I know better. All the best defensive player can do is take a basket or two or three away from me, but I must say that if you do that to a team's top scorer in a close game, it may be enough to cost his team the game. Just that much is important.

If you think about it, it's not really hard for a good scorer to average 20 points a game. That's five points a quarter, two baskets and a free-throw, say. On the pro level, 48-minute games, 12-minute quarters, that's a couple of points every five minutes. In the 40-minute college games and the 32-minute high school games it gets increasingly harder, of course, but if a player hustles, if he's aggressive, he doesn't have to be a gunner, he can play a balanced game and still get his share of points.

If he's aggressive he's going to be fouled and he's going to get some free-throws. If he's hustling he's going to get some loose balls, some follow-ups on missed shots, and some rebounds and tips. And if he looks for his

Here, in practice, I hook a short one over Jim McMillian, who got his hand up to try to deflect the ball off course. (Photography, Inc.)

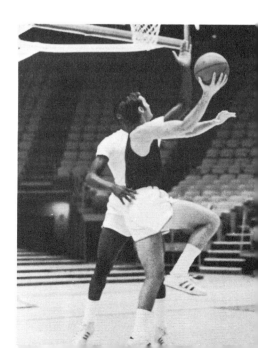

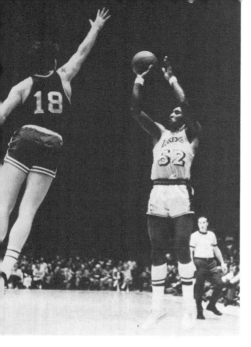

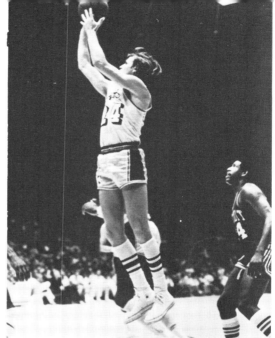

Happy Hairston (above left), Keith Erickson (above right), and Gail Goodrich (below) fire away. (Photography, Inc.)

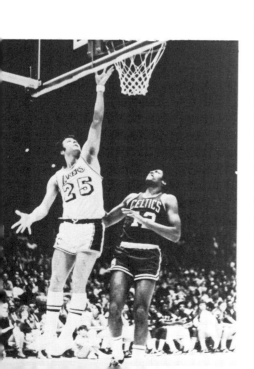

shots and shoots with reasonable accuracy he'll get his normal share of hoops. The better scorers will average around 30 points. Much more than that may be a bit suspect. It would seem to show that a fellow is taking too many shots, is taking too much on himself, perhaps is neglecting the rest of his game, although on some teams, without many good shooters, it may be asked of a fellow.

Here we should draw a distinction between a great shooter and a great scorer. There are fellows who are great scorers who are not great pure shooters. They are usually very aggressive fellows who have a knack of getting open for shots and are always going for the basket. Rick Barry is like this. He himself will tell you he's not a great shooter, although on some of his hard nights he sure looks like one. But, mainly, Rick goes for the basket. Elgin Baylor was another. Elgin might have been a great pure shooter had he shot normal shots, but I don't think Elg ever shot a normal shot in his life. He had incredible control of his body in the air and usually made driving, twisting shots which thrilled the crowd, often spinning the ball up from awkward positions with "English." In his best years, Elg seldom averaged better than

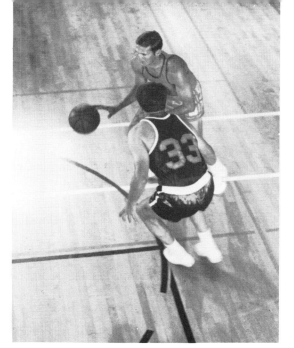

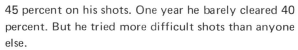

45 percent on his shots. One year he barely cleared 40 percent. But he tried more difficult shots than anyone else.

Another example of a scorer rather than a shooter is the big center who scores most of his baskets going up and shooting down at the basket from in close and getting a lot of tips. Although Wilt Chamberlain was fairly effective with a fadeaway shot from 10 to 15 feet for some seasons, he basically was not a good pure shooter but used his great size and strength to muscle in close and dunk the ball. The same goes for Walt Bellamy. Willis Reed has good pure shots and more variety. Kareem Jabbar has a lot more variety. He has a fine touch and is a great all-around shooter for a center. He hits about 65 percent of his free-throws. Wilt is lucky to hit 50 percent. These statistics don't lie. If they were superior pure shooters, they'd show it at the free-throw line. Some of these fellows, such as Wilt, hit a higher percentage from the field than from the free-throw line.

By "pure shooter" we mean a fellow who, without anyone bothering him, can stand out on the court in different places, shoot different shots, and hit a higher-than-average percentage. They have the mechanics mas-

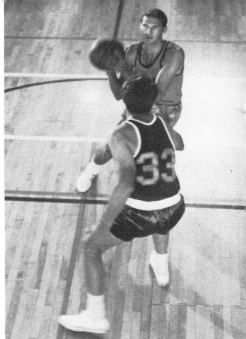

Driving on defender Rod Hundley, I dribble to the free-throw line, brake quickly, arresting my momentum and bringing the ball up, and go up to shoot a one-hand jumper over him before he can react sufficiently to stop me. (William Eastabrook for Sunkist Growers)

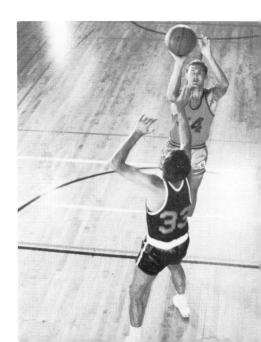

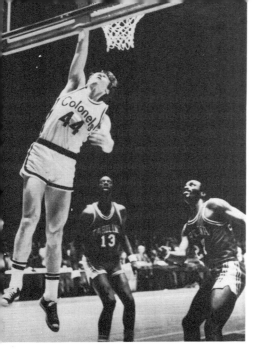

A brilliant rookie in the ABA in 1971, Dan Issel goes up to lay one in as Frank Card and Joe Caldwell watch. (Kentucky Colonels)

A powerful scorer and rebounder, Elvin Hayes, who as a Houston collegian led an upset over UCLA and had some memorable duels with Lew Alcindor, seems to be straining every muscle in his upper body as he goes up to try to lay the ball over the block attempt of LeRoy Ellis. (San Diego Rockets)

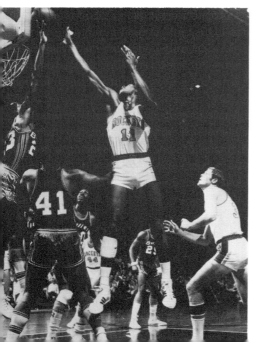

tered and a great touch. When you throw in a defender, however, and make the shooter work to get open for his best shots, then you introduce other elements which affect his ability to be a great scorer. We've all known fellows who were sharpshooters in practice but couldn't do it in games. I'm a good pure shooter with my jump-shot and my foul-shot. I'm more of a scorer with my other shots.

When you combine a great pure shooter with a great feel for scoring, then you've got a champion. In recent years, Adrian Smith, Flynn Robinson, Jerry Lucas, and Terry Dischinger have been fine pure shooters. Bob Love has turned into a great shooter under pressure. Oscar Robertson combines pure shooting ability with a scoring sense about as well as anyone. Willis Reed is a classic shooter for a center. Dave Bing, Charlie Scott, Spencer Haywood, and Bill Cunningham are good shooters and great scorers. Rick Barry, Artis Gilmore, Julius Erving, Dan Issel, and John Brisker are great scorers in the ABA.

How many points should a player score? He should score as many points as the number of shots he takes. Most will average less than 50 percent of their shots, but will make up for this with free-throws. Thus if a player takes ten shots he should not be satisfied with less than 10 points. If he takes twenty shots he should get 20 points. The good player should average success on 40 percent of his shots. If a player does not he should shoot less. He should take only those shots he can hit 40 percent with. He should practice until he can hit 70 to 75 percent of his free-throws. A reasonable goal is four of every ten field-shots, three of every four foul-shots.

It is a bit harder for a guard to score high because he usually shoots from further out and has to worry about getting back on defense. The forward shoots a lot from the corners, but he goes to the basket more than the guards and gets more follow-ups and tips. The center is right there at the basket, of course.

The player should look only for his good-percentage shots. If there are certain places on the court from which he can hit consistently, that's what he should look for. I have more good-percentage shots than most players. Elgin Baylor had more than anyone. He'd hit a far higher percentage of the shots he took than anyone else would. He could get you the difficult basket. Connie Hawkins and Julius Erving come close to his level. But few can, and few should try to emulate them.

A player can take some things from good shooters, but he can't copy them successfully. A player has a better chance at success if he develops his own natural, individual style. Look at the good shooters. Oscar Robertson differs from Earl Monroe, and both differ from Dick Barnett, who is extremely unorthodox, but all are successful. There is a lot of room for things to be done differently, yet successfully, in basketball, especially in shooting. It is not a game like golf, in which the individual apparently has to be locked in an awkward-feeling grip, stance, and swing to do well. The basketball player can find a comfortable style.

The player should take his shots when the right ones come up, but he should never shoot if there is someone he can pass to who is in position to take a better shot. This requires knowing yourself and your teammate. You have to make these decisions fast. Hesitation hurts. Sometimes it's simple, of course. No matter what kind of shot you have, if a teammate is wide open under the basket he should be given the ball. In any event, build up your speed as you go along. Forget about the 24-second rule. Don't copy the pros in this respect. Don't rush. By the time you get to be a pro you'll be sure enough of your moves to meet the demands of the 24-second clock, or the ABA's 30-second clock.

Years ago players always used the backboard, banking shots in. This only adds another obstacle to accuracy, however. It's very difficult to angle a shot off the back-

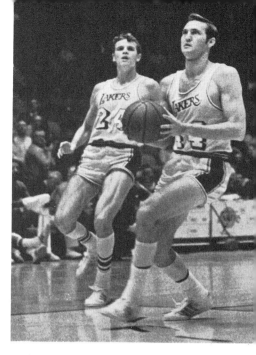

Ahead of the field on a fast-break, trailed by teammate Keith Erickson (above), I go in for a layup (below) as Bill Bradley moves into the picture in pursuit. (Photography, Inc.)

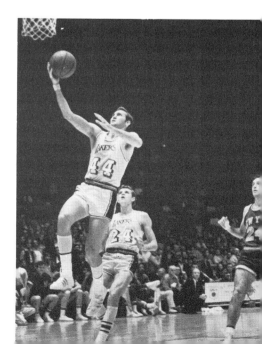

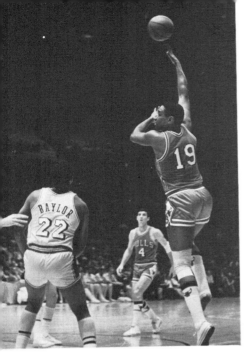

Driving out of a corner, forward Bob Boozer
shoots a classic hook while Elgin Baylor
(22) and Jerry Sloan (4) watch. (Photography, Inc.)

board in just the right place with just the right arc and
speed to send it through the hoop. Except for layups
and shots from difficult angles, shoot straight for the
basket. Shoot for one place on the rim all the time for
all shots. Most players will tell you to shoot for the back
of the rim, that if you do this, backspin will drop a lot
of soft shots in that otherwise would go astray. Personally, I shoot for the front of the rim, for what I can see,
and I can't see the back of the rim. I am shooting to
drop the ball just over the front of that rim. The important thing is to decide which part of the rim to aim at
and to use that part all the time. If you find you are
shooting short or long consistently, it is easy then to
make the adjustments.

Certain things are constant. The player should find a
relaxed position and develop a fluid motion. The younger and weaker the player, the less relaxed and fluid he
will be. But as he matures he will find he can be relaxed
and fluid within his own style. He should follow through
on all his shots, though the nature of the follow-through
may vary with the different shots. His shooting hand
should be centered to the basket while he is shooting.
His wrist should be relaxed, almost limp. The ball should
come off his fingers with natural spin, a natural backspin. The amount of rotation depends on his follow-
through. The longer the shot, usually, the less spin. He
should find the arc that works for him and keep it constant on all his shots. He should find the speed that
works for him and keep that constant.

Within these constants there are a few varieties. For
instance, most players will tell you to hold the ball in
your fingertips while shooting. They say your palm
should not come in contact with the ball. I think you get
a better feel of the ball, you get better balance with it
while it is in your hands, and you have more control of
it and can shoot it with greater strength if you hold it
against the pads of your hands. It still comes off your
fingertips when you shoot it. Frankly, I think more play-

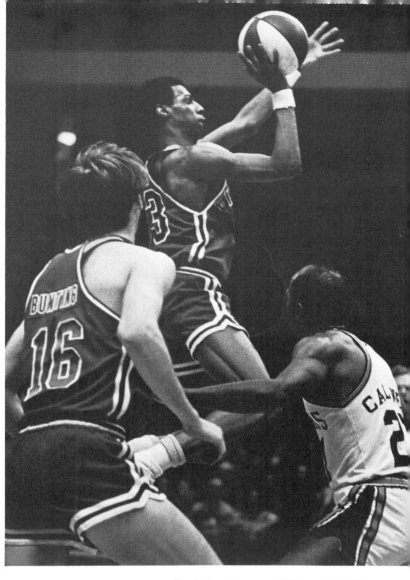

The ball on the pads of his hands, Charlie Scott, ABA rookie sensation in 1971, goes high for a picture-perfect one-hand jumper with Bill Bunting (16) and Joe Caldwell observing. (Austin Saunders for Virginia Squires)

ers hold the ball on the pads than will admit it. Watch them closely and you'll see this. The player should experiment and find what feels most comfortable and works best for him, and stick to it.

Another thing is the arc of the shot. Still another is the speed of it. I shoot flatter but softer than most. This varies tremendously with the individual. A high arc is very showy but extremely difficult to control. Most

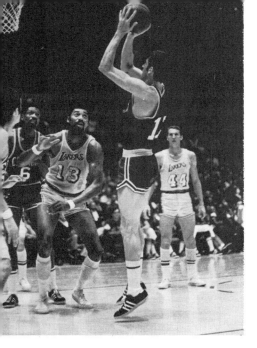

John Havlicek, a tireless super-scorer who is not a pure shooter but knows where the basket is, starts a one-hander with Wilt, Bill Russell, and a flat-footed West watching. (Photography, Inc.)

I shoot a jumper over Gus Johnson. (Photography, Inc.)

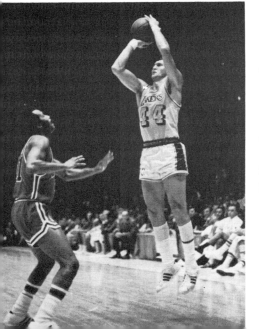

players preach a higher arc than I use, but all agree that the higher you go the less accurate you get. Within reason, you want enough height so that the ball comes down through the basket. Obviously, a perfectly flat shot will bounce off the rim. The flatter the shot, the less of the basket you seem to have to shoot at. But I have found that I am most accurate with a flat shot. As I get tired I tend to shoot harder and higher and lose accuracy. Sometimes, without realizing it, I try to compensate for increasing weariness.

Generally, all good players will tell you to try for a soft shot, the softer the better. It will tend to hang on the rim and drop in even if it does not have perfect accuracy. The harder the shot the more it tends to bounce away. But, strange as it sounds until you think about it, the younger and weaker you are the harder it is to shoot soft. The more effort it takes to get the ball up to the basket, the harder you tend to shoot it. With maturity you gain control over the ball, which enables you to send it up softly.

Oscar Robertson has an extremely soft shot. So does Lou Hudson. Sam Jones shot a soft shot. Yet, John Havlicek has had a lot of success with a much harder shot. Elg shot hard and often very flat. Sometimes he seemed to bang line-drives at the basket, but they went in. In any event, the player can only experiment with his, seeking the softest shot, the most gradual arc he can control, until he finds what works best for him. The important thing is, once he finds the right combination he should stick to it. You should not practice and use two entirely different shots. That is, you should practice and shoot set-shots and jump-shots and hooks and whatever it is you want to use, but the speed and arc should remain fairly constant from shot to shot, with only slight variations according to the type of shot.

If you find that you are undershooting or overshooting, adjust your speed. While you are finding your way, lean toward overshooting instead of undershooting.

Overshooting, your misses at least can often be re-bounded by yourself or your teammates. Undershooting, your misses most often will fall in a defender's hands. If you find your shots are going too much to the right or left, you are applying too much pressure to the ball on the opposite side.

Generally, shooters are made, not born. It takes a certain amount of natural strength, reflexes, and timing to shoot well, but most shooting skills can be developed with practice. It certainly is a skill you can practice alone or with a friend. Even if you are not playing regularly you can build up your shooting skills in prac-tice. Bill Sharman always says that shooting is a memory skill. You find your best rhythm and use your muscles in the same way again and again, gaining a groove, building up your confidence. If you do it exactly the same way every time it will work the same way every time. Proof of this lies in free-throw shooting. Bunny Levitt, who used to give exhibitions, once sank 499 in a row before he missed one, then 371 more before he missed another.

Beyond the free-throw shot, the best shot is the closest shot you can get. The layup is the ideal shot. The player should miss very few of these. Rarely should the player shoot from more than 20 feet away. He should work to build up his range, but 20 feet is a reasonable limit to set. Beyond that, most shooters are pressing. However, the ABA favors outside shooters with a line curving across the court, from 22 feet in the corners to 25 feet in the center, beyond which shooters get 3 points for a basket instead of 2. Some players develop startling accuracy from this range. In 1971, George Leh-mann hit an astonishing 154 of 382 for .403. In 1972, Glenn Combs of Utah hit 103 of 254 for .406. Consider that these players got 3 points instead of 2 for each and yet sustained a 40-percent accuracy level and you can see they did quite a job for their teams.

Building up the greatest range will help a player in many ways. The farther he shoots from the basket the

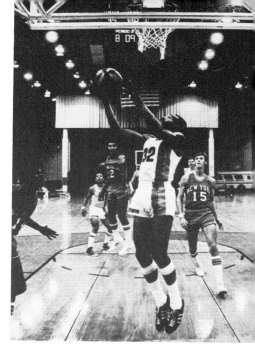

Larry Jones, record-setting ABA scorer, goes up for a reverse layup. (Jay Spencer for Floridians)

Catching everyone flat-footed, Archie Clark comes from behind the basket to lay up a backhander. Watching, left to right, are Rick Roberson, yours truly, Jim Washington, Willie McCarter, and Keith Erickson. (Pho-tography, Inc.)

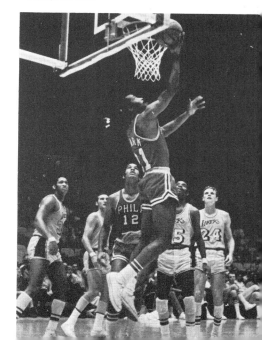

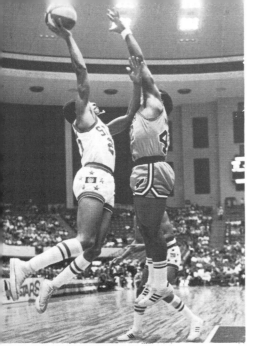

Springy little Donnie Freeman one-hands one in ABA game. (Paul Barker for Deseret *News*)

The follow-through form of little Mack Calvin, the 6-foot flash from USC who made good in the ABA, is shown here after a one-hand attempt. (Floridians)

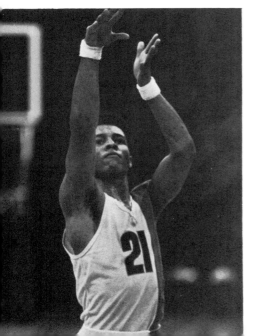

less defensive pressure there is. The greater the reputation he gains for long shots the more the defense will move up on him, making it easier for him to drive around his defender and opening up the middle. And the sooner he can put up a reasonable shot the better it will be if his team needs points in a hurry toward the game's end. However, again the key thing is that you should shoot only those shots, and from that range that you can handle with around 40 percent accuracy.

Another thing a player should build up is an ability to shoot layups and hooks with either hand. I learned to use my left hand as a pro. I really wish I'd learned earlier.

"Little" players like Gail Goodrich, Calvin Murphy. Flynn Robinson, Guy Rodgers, Nate Archibald, Len Wilkens, Mack Calvin, Bill Melchionni, Larry Brown, and others who became pro stars, although 6-2 or shorter, did so mainly because they had the versatility to shoot from long-range or penetrate defenses with drives, to dribble and shoot with both hands, to make the most of every weapon available to them.

Fakes are an important weapon. A player must master a variety of fakes. He must use his feet, his hands, his shoulders, his eyes, and his head to taunt the defender and throw him off stride.

However, I think players waste energy and waste the value of fakes with too many of them. A few good fakes mixed up over the course of a game are all a player needs. One good fake is all he needs before making each move, and many times he does not even need this. Look in one direction, then go in the other. Shake the ball in one direction, then go in the other. Step in one direction, then go the other way. Keep it subtle. Don't make it so bold that it's obvious you're trying to draw attention to it. But, sometimes, look in one direction, then go in that direction. Shake the ball one way, then go that way. And so forth. Mix 'em up. But use fakes conservatively. Never get typed. And save your best moves for when they are needed the most.

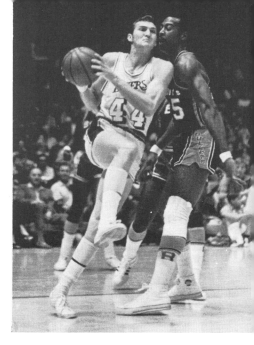

The most important thing in shooting is the speed with which you get your shot off. The defenders don't know when you're going to shoot and the type of shot you're going to take, and the quicker you do it the less chance they have to react. This, more than anything else, is the secret to any success I've had. When I am going to shoot I never hesitate. Usually, I take a jump-shot. Sometimes I drive. I'm not among the fastest players in pro ball, but I get some of the quickest starts.

I'm only 6-3 but have extremely long arms that compensate somewhat for my lack of height, but by pro standards I'm really a short player. Nor do I jump as high as many. I actually shoot before I reach the peak of my jump, unlike most shooters. I get rid of the ball fast, which takes practice. There is no point in rushing your shot to the degree where you can't control it. But the quicker your moves and the greater your control, the better off you will be. A split-second advantage in quickness is worth a dozen fakes. Within 20 feet your best fake usually is no fake. If there is a single sin I find in most players it is that they usually fake too much and waste themselves. Even if they fool their foe, they often have nothing left with which to use the advantage they've gained.

Learn not only the shots you can make with an acceptable degree of accuracy but the shots your particular defender can defend against best. If a man is tough to drive around, don't try to drive around him very often. If a fellow blocks a lot of your shots, increase the quickness of your shot, its speed, and its arc. Don't get discouraged when you have a shot blocked. This is a rapidly developing art in basketball. The shorter we are the more shots we're apt to have blocked. But if you do have a shot blocked, consider it your fault. Make whatever adjustments you can. And if you get an unreasonable number of shots blocked by a certain player, you're going to have to stop shooting within his range.

Master as many shots and as great a range and as

Driving hard and going up for the basket, I burst around the brilliant and vastly underrated veteran Gus Johnson. I seem to have lowered my shoulder, he seems to have taken a fixed position. Would you have called a foul? Which way? I don't believe one was called. (Photography, Inc.)

Coming around and under, I lay one in from behind as Walt Hazzard leans on me. (Photography, Inc.)

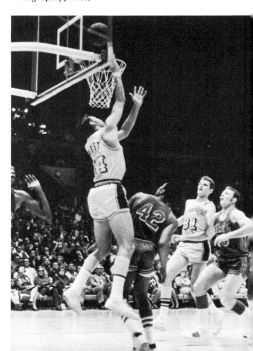

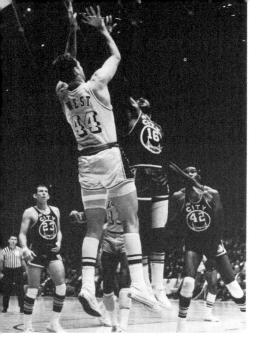

The one-hand jump-shot at the instant of release, just as my guide hand falls from the ball. Al Attles is going up with me here while Jeff Mullins (23) and Nate Thurmond (42) watch. I am giving it a little fadeaway here to free me from the intense defensive pressure. (Photography, Inc.)

much quickness as you can. Keep working. Most of the best players practice all the time. A lot of the great players play in pickup games during the off-season and they'll tell you they never stop improving. Keep stretching yourself. I couldn't go to my left for shots until I worked on it as a pro. I was an all-state player in high school and an all-American in college, but I hadn't come close to mastering important techniques until I got to pro ball, and even as an all-pro I find I am improving parts of my game every season. Sometimes you can get by with less, but the higher you go the more you'll need. And it's obvious that the more you have on any level, the better you'll do.

When I went into a shooting slump during the 1972 playoffs, it was very difficult to shake it. At first I could not put my finger on the problem. Almost everyone was giving me advice. I was even getting phone-calls, letters and telegrams from fans and it would have been easy to get mixed-up. Finally, I figured out that I wasn't getting properly set, and wasn't going straight up and coming straight down. I was rushing my shots and leaning forward a little. But once you become anxious and begin to press, once you lose confidence and begin to think through every move instead of moving naturally, it is hard to regain your touch. It proved that no matter how long you play and how successful you are, you can have problems. But if your game is fundamentally sound, you will find your way back to normal.

5. The Shots

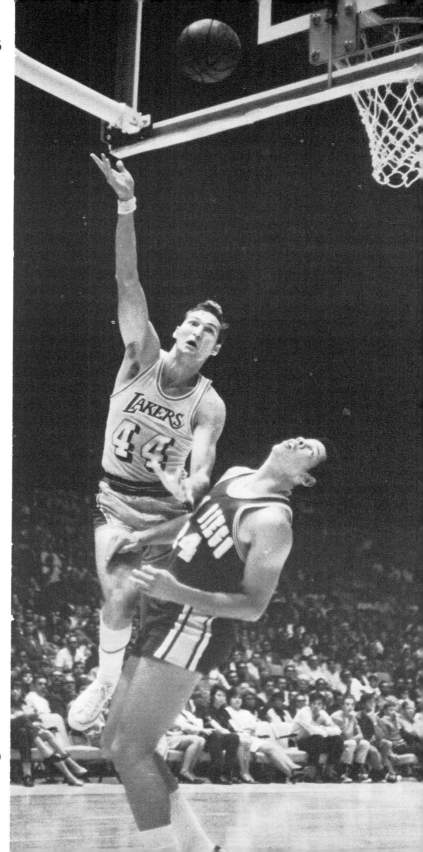

Running over a foe, who has closed off my path to a layup, I leap for a sort of in-close hook-shot. (Photography, Inc.)

THERE ARE almost as many shots in basketball as there are positions into which we can twist our bodies, arms, elbows, and hands. Whatever the shot you are taking, and whatever the mechanics of that particular shot, the things that will most determine its success are side-to-side accuracy, arc, and force.

If you put the 9-inch basketball directly in the center of the 18-inch hole, you have 4½ inches on either side to spare. Obviously, if you are 4½ inches or more off to either side the ball is going to bounce off the rim. If your shot is too flat it is going to bounce off the front or back rim. If it is soft enough, a shot that may be slightly off may "hang" on the rim and fall in.

The key factors are your stance, your body balance, your grip on the ball, the position of your arms, elbows, and hands, your footwork, your follow-through, and, throughout it all, your "feel" for the basket, how hard and how far and in which direction you shoot.

Basically, you should be relaxed and comfortable, with your body in balance and your style grooved. It is possible with a great sense of body-control to shoot off-balance shots successfully, as the Elgin Baylors and Connie Hawkins have proved, but there are not many like them, and even they will tell you that it is not the best way.

Essentially, every shot is like a free-throw, it can be grooved. Operating at top speed under defensive pressure and with the possibility that you should pass off always in your mind, all shots differ from free-throws. But they have in common the fact that, whatever the shot, if you practice it until you shoot it exactly the same way each time, you will become relaxed with it, become comfortable with it, and confident of it.

You must concentrate. This can be built up. You must bear down on the job at hand while shutting everything else from your mind—the crowd, parents in the stands, a girl in the stands, any personal problems you

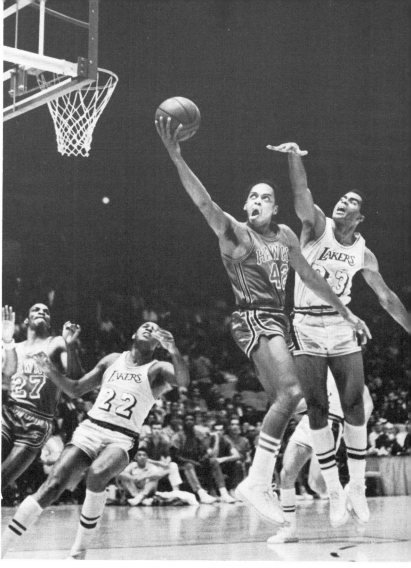

may have. And you must forget about statistics. You can't be thinking, "If I make this I'll have 10 points for the game." You can't be thinking, "I've missed three in a row, I have to make this one." Each move, each play, each shot, is new and different and demands your complete concentration.

You must see what your teammates are doing and what the defenders are doing, you must decide what you

Face contorted with the effort, body twisted, Walt Hazzard reaches back to attempt to shovel in a one-hand underhander as Tom Hawkins reaches in and Joe Caldwell and Elgin Baylor brake and come careening to a halt. (Photography, Inc.)

are going to do and you must do it. You must know the game situation. While you should never rush beyond reason, if you are behind with time running out you have to step up the pace, though never beyond your ability to control it. If a team is defending loosely and you can penetrate, go to the short game. If they are defending the basket closely, go to a longer game. Selecting your shots, you mix them up, but you pick those that work best for you and will work best in the particular situation.

No one is born with this knowledge. The more you play the more experienced you become. With experience your mind becomes a sort of computer. Whatever the situation, you have been there before. You don't have a lot of time to think out each move, each shot. You have to react. With experience, as each play develops, the possibilities will sort swiftly through the computer and you'll make the best possible selections.

The oldest shot in basketball is the two-hand set-shot, but it is seldom used these days. Even so, it remains basic because the youngest beginners often do not have the strength to take other shots as well and because it is a fundamental shot from which many others have grown. The longer the distance the better a shot it is. You have the force of both hands, both arms, and your entire body behind the shot. Since few can shoot it well nowadays, and since defenses pick up a player quickly, there is little call for the two-hand set-shot on higher levels.

Shooting this shot, you square your body to the basket. If you are shooting from a side, you take an angle so your body remains directly behind the flight of the ball. Seek a comfortable stance. Do not spread your feet too wide. When Rochester won the NBA title back in 1951, its two best shooters were two-hand set-shooters, Bobby Wanzer and Bob Davies. Wanzer kept his feet together, feeling he could get more thrust and power when he unflexed his knees upward. Davies, however was successful with his feet slightly spread. When I take this shot, which I rarely do, I spread my feet about 12 inches.

Bend slightly at the knees and lean slightly forward over the ball. The farther out you are, the more force you need and the more you should bend, but never bend so far that you lose balance and tilt forward. Bending the knees compensates for leaning over the ball and tends to keep you in balance. Shooting from the side, I tend to put the foot on that side slightly ahead of the other foot.

Hold the ball chest-high. Hold your elbows in to your sides. Your elbows are cocked. Hold the ball with your hands on the rear sides of the ball, fingers spread, thumbs to the rear of the ball. Hold the ball about a foot in front of your body. Again, the pads of my hands are in contact with the ball. Many will tell you that only your fingers should touch the ball. If that works for you, fine, but I have found that most players actually touch the ball with their pads and I think that I have a better feel of the ball and more control of it in this way.

Sight the target over the top of the ball, bend at the knees a bit more to coil for the thrust, point your elbows up a bit to coil for the thrust, which tends to bring the ball back, begin to shoot by uncoiling from your knees, then your elbows, finally your wrists as you thrust your arms forward. You may actually give a little jump, or, at least, a slight lift off the court, as you follow through, but never pitch forward. The ball spins off your fingers and you follow through straight at the basket, but as your arms reach their full extension, the natural thrust has turned your hands outward to the sides.

This shot can also be taken as an over-the-head shot. The main difference is that the ball is held either over the top of the head or at forehead height. The same fundamentals apply except that the elbows are held higher, the arms are tilted back at a 45-degree angle, and the

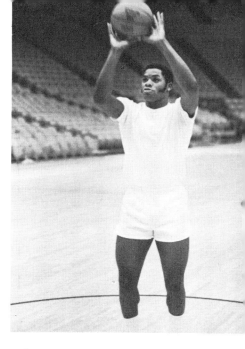

Demonstrating two-hand set-shot form, Jim McMillian lets one go. (Photography, Inc.)

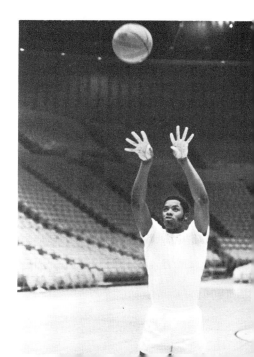

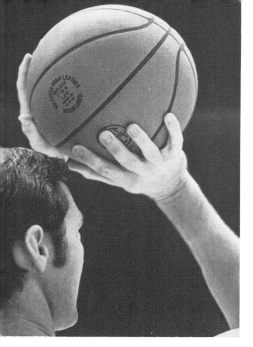

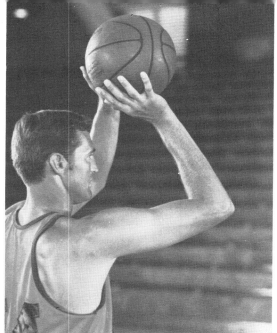

The one-hand shot from overhead position is demonstrated on these two pages: from the pads of my hand flush on the ball through to the final limp-hand follow-through, hand pointing at the basket. (Photography, Inc.; William Eastabrook for Sunkist Growers)

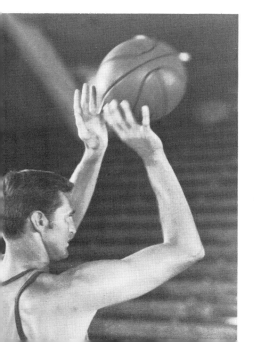

shot is taken more with arm- and wrist-snap than with an uncoiling from the knees.

The advantage of this shot is that it is quick and can be snapped over tall defenders, especially under tight defensive pressure, such as in the corners, where defenders tend to press. Furthermore, the defender must raise his hands to protect against it and is vulnerable to a swift shift into a drive; also, the shooter can snap a quick pass to the pivotman. But there are also disadvantages. You lose some control of the ball, you lose some potential force with the chest-high shot, and since you are standing erect with your arms held high, you lose time bringing the ball down and your body and legs are not in good position for a quick drive. However, this shot is a good weapon and in today's game is probably more valuable for the more advanced player than the two-hand chest-high set, though it stems from that one, which must be mastered first.

Carl Braun, a former New York Knick, and Larry Friend, a former Cal player and pro with the Knicks and Los Angeles Jets of the short-lived American Basketball League of the early 1960's, were two who featured the overhead set-shot. Friend became the best 3-point shoot-

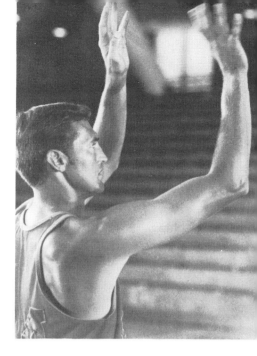

er in the ABL with it. Wallace "Wah Wah" Jones, former Kentucky all-American and pro star, is another who had great success with this shot. In recent seasons, Richie Guerin used this shot extensively.

The one-hand set shot is an outgrowth of the two-hand chest-high set. Some say you have greater control of the two-hand set because you have two hands controlling the ball. Others say you have better control of the one-hand set for the same reason, because you don't have a second hand to go wrong. Take your pick. I lean to the second theory. I think it is easier to do everything exactly right with one hand, with one elbow, with one arm, than with two.

The body position and posture for the one-hand set is similar to that for the two-hand set. The hand position, however, differs greatly. Your feet are spread shoulder-width, the foot under your shooting hand a few inches ahead of the other foot, your shooting-side knee bent less than the other. Your elbow is held well up, pointed almost at the basket. Your wrist is cocked and your hand is flat and directly under the ball with your fingers spread but at a relaxed width. I hold the ball higher than for a one-hand shot, more like my jump-shot—just over my head.

Again, I hold the ball on the pads of my hand. So does Oscar Robertson. Oscar, who has a masterfully grooved one-hand shot, uses an extreme style in that his elbow is held higher, his wrist flexed back farther than any other shooter I know. He sometimes seems about to push the ball directly overhead. Jerry Lucas has amazing accuracy with a high arch one-hand set-shot that makes him look like a shot-putter, but he was tremendous with it at times in the 1972 playoffs.

As with most shooters, my hand is angled slightly toward the basket. You push the ball up and forward, but the force of the release comes more from the snapping of your elbow and wrist than from an arm thrust. The ball comes off your fingertips, giving it backspin and

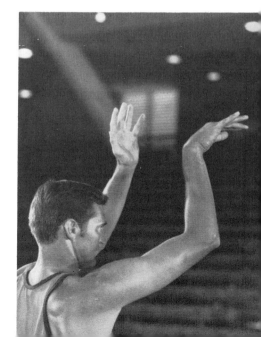

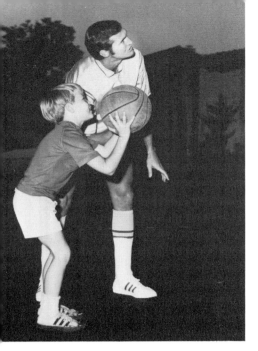

Attempting a one-hand shot, my son Mark must use all his might. A two-hand set might be better for him. (Photography, Inc.)

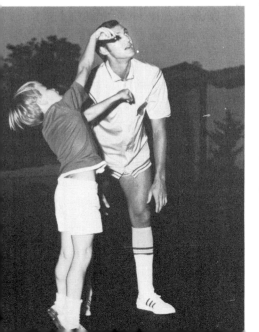

making it soft. And as it does you are rising up to your toes, giving a little spring, not a jump. Thus your body is slightly behind the shot and there is a smooth interrelated series of body movements.

Never give any shot excessive spin, no matter how fancy the ball looks as it rotates through the air. You are not throwing baseball pitches. You want the ball to go straight with soft backspin. You do not deliberately add spin. As it comes off your fingertips, it will do so with soft backspin.

Too flat a shot is too easily blocked, but try to find a natural arc that is not too pronounced. You start from a semiseated position. Never thrust forward too sharply, which would cause you to lunge as you shoot. Follow all the way through to a full extension of the arm with your wrist and fingers limp and angled in the direction of the basket. As you settle back to the court you have not gone forward but have returned to your standing position with your feet in their original position.

Always keep your head still, your eyes squared on the target. Don't bob your head up and down, looking at the ball and following the shot. Keep your eyes on the basket. The ball is held chest-high and as it comes up and over it passes to the side of your face forehead-high before being brought forward. Carry it as high as feels comfortable. Oscar carries it high. I aim for just over the front of the rim. Most good shooters miss short more than long.

Use your free hand alongside the ball until you begin your shot. This protects the ball and gives you greater control of it. It must drop off as you begin to shoot, however. Held too long against the ball, it will push your motion off-center. It is important that your elbow stay in and your arm follow a straight path, and that your cocked wrist and hand remain straight behind the ball, centered to the target. Repetitious practice will groove this. Any wandering of your elbow or twisting of your wrist or hand, any indirect arm thrust will tend to shove the ball right or left. If the ball is off-center, your elbow has been too far out or too far in, or you have twisted your arm, hand, or wrist in delivery.

This is just as good a shot as a jump-shot. It is a surer shot. As you advance into more intense competition and tighter guarding, you will have to turn more and more to the jump-shot off this basic shot, but whenever you can get off a standing one-hand set do so, as it is perhaps the most solid shot in today's arsenal. Gail Goodrich is a good example of a great one-hand set-shot specialist. Jack Kent Cooke says he seems to float feathers at the basket, Gail's shot is so soft.

The most famous name that endures from early basketball, Hank Luisetti came out of Stanford and the Far West to revolutionize basketball with the one-hand shot, starting with the standing one-hand set and going on to the running one-hand set and the jump-shot. In 1936 he went into Madison Square Garden and his shooting ended Long Island University's 43-game winning streak. Less than two years later he went into Pittsburgh and scored 50 points in a single game against Duquesne, an incredible and never-to-be-forgotten performance in an era when whole teams seldom scored that many points in a game.

He developed the shot to the point where he took it off the drive from just beyond the foul circle. He never played pro ball, which was in its disorganized infancy at the time, but went on to service and AAU ball. In 1950 he ranked just behind George Mikan in the "player of the half-century" voting, a rare honor because he had been retired for more than a decade.

Until Luisetti, players either shot two-hand sets with their feet planted or driving layups. He may have been the single most revolutionary player ever, ranking with George Mikan, who popularized the hook-shot; Bob Cousy, who popularized fancy dribbling and passing; and Bill Russell, who revolutionized defensive play. Luisetti was the forerunner of Joe Fulks, who with his acrobatic one-handers was the first great scorer in pro ball and was the forerunner of myself and all the other one-hand

Oscar Robertson, the greatest all-around backcourt player I've faced, demonstrates his individual style on the one-hand set-shot he shoots from the field and the free-throw line. His elbow, pointed at the basket, is thrust almost in front of his face (he seems to sight through his elbow), the ball is held high and on the pads of his hand, with his wrist cocked far more than most. (Photography, Inc.)

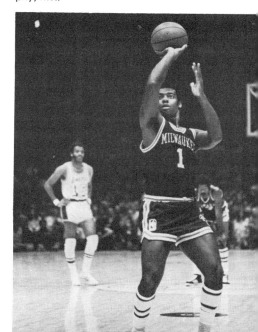

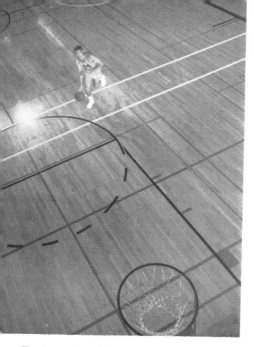
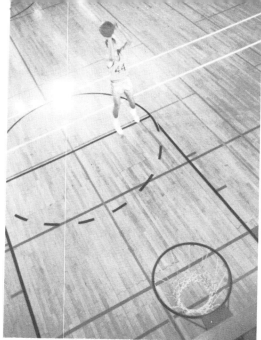

The jump-shot off a dribble from the free-throw line. I come down in the same spot from which I jumped, watching the flight of the ball all the way. (William Eastabrook for Sunkist Growers)

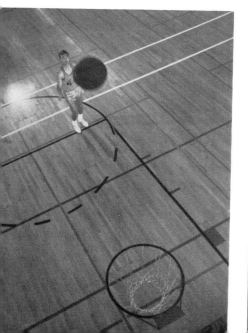
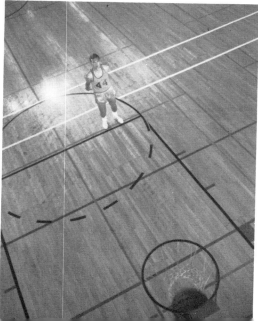

jump-shot specialists who have dominated the game in
recent years.

The one-hand jump-shot is shot almost the same as
the one-hand set-shot, except that it comes at the conclusion of motion and is taken with a jump into the air.
In this way it can be shot more quickly, the ball is released higher, and it is harder to defend or block. Obviously, since it is taken while moving and jumping,
there is a greater chance of error than in the standing
set-shot, but we have been able to groove this shot. It
can be shot with as much accuracy as any shot, aside
from the free-throw and layup, and more than any other
shot is responsible for the fabulous increase in scoring.

It is usually taken off a dribble, short or long, and
sometimes off a fake. The key thing is that the defender
does not know when you are going up. If you do not tip
off your move, if you go up quick, and if you have a
quick release, you have a tremendous edge on any defender. If you are driving in to the middle you must have
a quick enough shot and a high enough arc so that the
big center can't bat it back down your throat. One of
the ways big centers get the job done, however, even
when they do not block the shot, is to force the jump-
shooter into such an unnaturally high arc that he misses
his shot.

In shooting a jumper off a dribble, make your last
dribble hard so that you can pick up the ball high. If you
are leaning right or left or forward or backward when
you shoot, your chances of success are greatly dimin-
ished. Go straight up.

The legs must be synchronized in this shot more than
in most. The biggest fault with most players attempting
this shot is that they attempt to jump too high, forcing
their move and losing their rhythm and body-control.
Jump only as high as you can comfortably while keeping

the body under control. For most players this may not be more than 6 to 12 inches off the court, but this adds a lot of height. Some players naturally spring higher without losing control of their bodies, and this is an asset but is not the most critical aspect to successful jump-shooting.

The act of jumping sends some force and thrust into your shot, but don't let it overpower your shot. You still get the strength of the shot from up top, from the basic elbow-snap and wrist-snap. Aside from the fundamentals of keeping your arm, wrist, and hand straight-on to the target, I believe the most critical factor in controlling a jump-shot is a straight up-and-down jump. To this end, in practice, I have always taken note of the precise position of my feet and the precise place on the court they occupied when I went up so I could see if I came down in the same place. I believe it is vital to come down in your footsteps. You can't keep looking up and down, but once you get an awareness of this, you will feel it. Nothing causes jump-shots to miss more often than a body thrust that sends you forward or backward or to one side. Know how to set yourself properly.

Carry the ball in both hands until you go up, let your other hand drop off and raise the ball as you jump, cocking your wrist. Sight on the basket as you are going up,

The position of the feet in the jump-shot is shown on these two pages. Here I begin to brake at the foul line, come to a halt, bend at the knees for the jump, and go up and come down. It is an optical illusion that the jump has carried me past the foul line. In the last picture you see I have come down only slightly ahead of my take-off spot. I'd have preferred to come down in my exact footsteps. (William Eastabrook for Sunkist Growers)

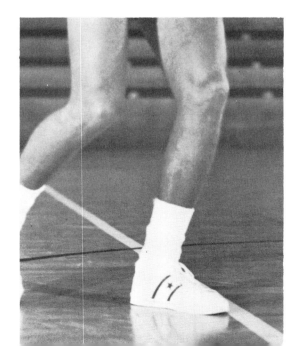

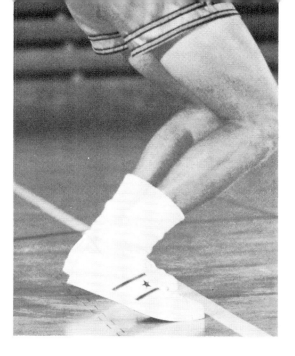 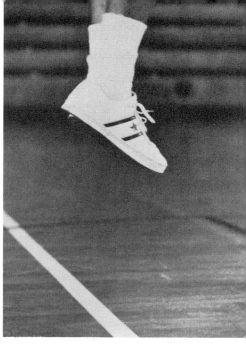

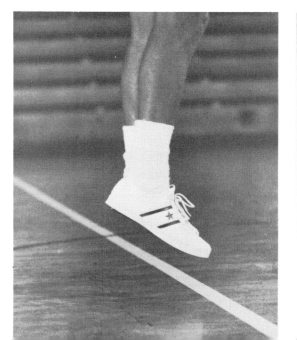 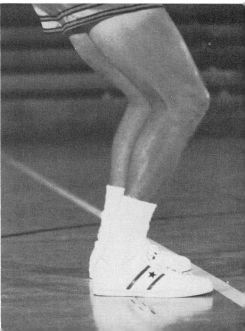

not after you have reached the top of your jump. Try to shoot near or at the very peak of your jump, not on the way up or the way down. There is a split-second there when you have reached the peak of your jump when you will feel as though you are hanging there, and it is in this split-second that most feel the shot is best taken although I, personally, do shoot a bit sooner.

The arm must be straight with your elbow under the ball. The wrist is cocked and the ball flows off the fingertips at the release. As you move into position for the jump, stop on the foot closest to the basket, come to a two-foot stop to arrest your motion, then stand in an erect position. No matter how hard you are coming or in which directions you throw fakes, you must still go straight up and come straight down when you shoot. Keep your head up and follow through to the extended-arm, limp-wrist, limp-hand, limp-fingers position. The ball is released well above the head as the arm reaches its full extension up and forward. Don't get the ball too far in front of you or too close to your body.

It is extremely difficult to shoot this shot properly from a standing position without some movement. It is usually best to take at least one dribble, plant the feet firmly, and go up with both feet at the same time instead of favoring one foot or the other. Practice this shot over and over again until you are completely comfortable with it. The younger and weaker and less experienced you are the more awkward and uncomfortable this shot will feel, but you should work on it until it is as basic to you as throwing a baseball.

Players such as Joe Caldwell and Dave Bing easily reach tremendous heights without any apparent effort for their jump-shots. It is a help, but it would be a hindrance if they went up higher than they could with full control. Mack Calvin, Charlie Scott, and Donnie Free-

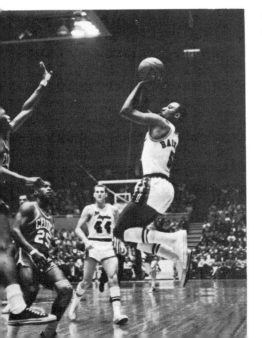

"Fall back, baby," when Dick Barnett, leaping with his legs tucked under him, goes up for a jumper that will wind up with Dick fading away at the finish. Dick's falling-backward jumpers are unorthodox but effective. (Photography, Inc.)

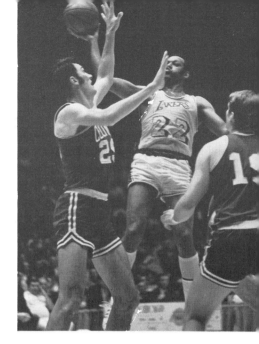

man are good ones. Dick Barnett shoots the most unorthodox jump-shot. It is a "fallaway" or "fadeaway" jumper. He falls back, seemingly off-balance as he shoots. It became his trademark. Sure of himself, he used to shout "Fall back, baby" as he shot, suggesting that all should go back on defense instead of following the shot as it was going in. I guess he still does it. But Barnett actually is not out of balance, because the shot comes naturally to him, and he has great control of his body while shooting it.

I don't recommend others to shoot Dick's way—I don't think he would—but it works for him and could work for others. It has a great advantage in that he is going away from the defender as he shoots, so it is a difficult shot to guard.

Actually, I have good jump-shooting form, and this is one of the areas in which the young player might wish to watch me. I have good spring in my legs and unusually long arms for a man my height and, more than anything else, I have quickness, all of which has enabled me to go up quick, get the ball higher than most people my size, and get the shot off quicker than most players.

Many players have developed variations off the basic jump-shot. Under tremendous defensive pressure in crowds, Connie Hawkins and Earl Monroe can contort their bodies, twist, and get off incredible shots while seemingly suspended high in the air. Baylor probably was the greatest exponent of the twisting one-hander shot off balance. The fact is, he had such control of his body, his arms, and his hands, and such a feel for the basket, that he really was not off balance.

Connie Hawkins can do it. He has the biggest hands I've ever seen, long arms, and incredible body control. I think he more than Elg sometimes tries shots that are beyond him, but he sure makes some spectacular ones.

The off-balance shot is misnamed in the case of its leading specialist, Elgin Baylor, who has complete control of his body and hands in the air and is able to take shots others wouldn't dare attempt. Here, above, he moves the ball around in one hand while "hanging" to find a path to shoot over Henry Finkel (29) and Don Nelson (19), and, below, he flips the ball basketward off a ballet step as Happy Hairston and Lou Hudson, left, watch. (Photography, Inc.)

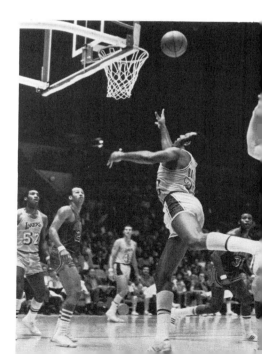

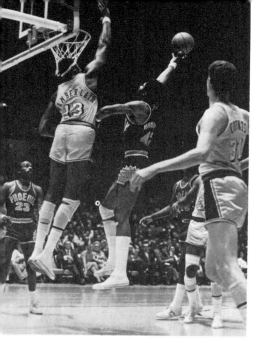

Twisting around Wilt, Connie Hawkins reaches a long arm and spins the ball off his long fingertips toward the basket. Art Harris is watching at the left and Mel Counts is moving up at the right. (Photography, Inc.)

So does Monroe, who is a 6-3 guard and is one of the exciting players I'd pay to see play. Like 6-5 Elg, most of these fellows developed this style to make up for being defensed by bigger men.

You can't teach this sort of thing. You can practice it to some extent. Mainly, you develop it off the sound fundamental shot. Necessity becomes the mother of invention. You don't start with this sort of shot. You begin with the basic jumper. As you gain experience you may experiment with different shots that will get you out of tight spots. The real danger in these shots is that most of them are forced, and you should never force a shot.

If you don't have a good shot, your good shot, you shouldn't take a shot. If you can shoot unorthodox shots without forcing them, if you can be consistently effective with them, fine, welcome to an exclusive club, but if it's beyond you, forget it. These shots are only sensational in the hands of experts. They look ludicrous in the hands of most players. Trying to look sensational, most players look bad.

The hook-shot, though showy, is not really an unorthodox shot but a basic shot that every player should master. I think George Mikan probably did more to popularize this shot than any other player. He was 6-10, 245 pounds, and tremendously strong. I understand he was not a graceful giant in all respects, but he had a graceful hook-shot. He averaged 22 points a game through a ten-year pro career, averaged 27 or 28 points a game at his peak, and led the Lakers, then in Minneapolis, to five pennants and five playoff titles in the late 1940's and early 1950's.

Neil Johnston and Easy Ed Macauley were others of his era who had great hook-shots. Clyde Lovellette was another, and Sweetwater Clifton and Goose Tatum from the Harlem Globetrotters. The shot simply is not used much today, which is a shame because it is almost impossible to defend against. However, Kareem Abdul-Jabbar has a classic hook, as does Willis Reed.

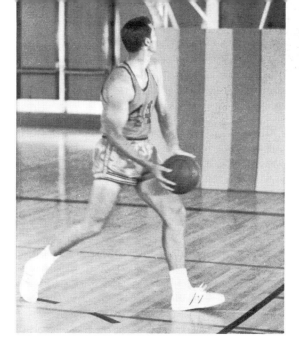

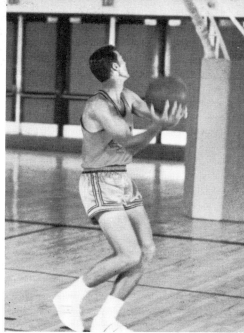

My way to shoot a hook shot—turning my back to the basket, then striding left, pointing my shoulder at the hoop, and bringing the ball around and about 6 inches from my face, with my hand pointed toward the basket at the finish. (William Eastabrook for Sunkist Growers)

Essentially, the hook is a center's shot, but Baylor, Cliff Hagan, and Tom Heinsohn were forwards who were enormously effective with hooks from the corner, and Bob Cousy was a guard who made great use of it, especially while sweeping cross-court from just behind the foul circle. I wish I had mastered it. It looks difficult, but it can be grooved until it is consistently effective. You can make a good pass off of a hook. The hook-shot is not enough by itself. Billy McGill, who led the nation's collegians in scoring with it while at Utah, probably had as classic a hook-shot as anyone ever, but he didn't have enough to go with it and bounced around the pros for years without attaining stardom.

The player turns his back partly to the basket and brings the ball, held in both hands, to his hip or below. Some players stride away from the basket as they start the shot, then stride toward the basket as they shoot, giving them a sort of rocking motion. I believe the step away from the basket is unnecessary. I stride more to the side. Shooting a right-handed hook, point your left shoulder at the basket and stride with your left foot. Keeping your head up, turned to the basket, bring the ball out, away from the basket, almost to the full exten-

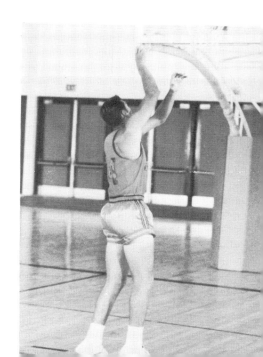

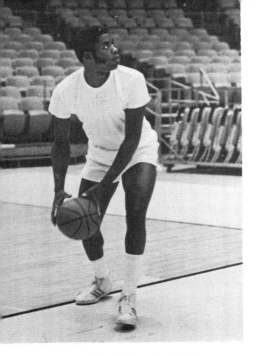

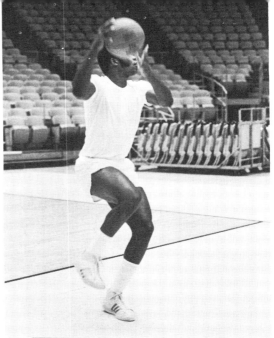

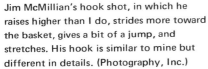

Jim McMillian's hook shot, in which he raises higher than I do, strides more toward the basket, gives a bit of a jump, and stretches. His hook is similar to mine but different in details. (Photography, Inc.)

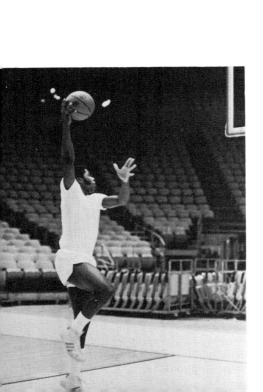

sion of your hand, dropping your helping hand from it. As you pivot to your left, twisting around to turn your upper torso toward the basket, as you stride, bring your arm in a wide arc along the side of your face, not over your head. As your left leg pushes down, your right leg is drawn up high, knee bent. You release the ball at the peak of your swing and your arm continues through to face-level in your follow-through. Your hand is aimed at the basket at all times.

Because the ball is moved at the greatest distance from the defender between you and the basket, it is a difficult shot for him to frustrate. And because you never see the ball while you are shooting it, you must work on it until the motion that will drop the ball into the basket consistently is completely comfortable and grooved. It is not an entirely natural motion and it takes practice to get the timing right, but it is a tremendously useful shot that is not used as much as it should be.

Aside from Jabbar and Willis Reed, Nate Thurmond and Bob Rule are others who have superior hook-shots. Wilt Chamberlain never developed one he uses consistently, preferring to muscle in close or shoot a fadeaway

jumper. The criticism of his fadeaway is that it carries
him away from the backboard and out of the play. One
virtue of the hook-shot is that with the thrust of the leg
toward the basket, the player's momentum sends him
toward the backboard, following his own shot, and toward whatever play may develop from it. Wilt also has a
most unusual shot, a "finger roll," in which from fairly
far in front of the basket he reaches to it and lets the
ball roll off his fingers toward it. It takes a man of his
over-7-foot height and tremendous reach to use such a
showy shot with any degree of effectiveness.

Somewhere in-between the jump-shot and the layup
are the driving one-handers used by many big men. Most
of these are more basic and less varied than the showy
shots of an Elgin Baylor or a Connie Hawkins, but they
also require great body-control. Bob Pettit, who seemed
to get to the basket through sheer determination, used
to bang in these driving, short jumpers. Rick Barry, who
is a deadly shooter from within 15 feet, is another who
finds holes to blast through and pops in these shorties.
He says growing up he copied Baylor and mastered a
wide variety of driving shots. Jim McMillian has great
body control on driving shots.

Spencer Haywood, who has enormous hands and
great spring and strength, is another who can get through
and drop in bombs from close range. Julius Erving and
Dan Issel are others. Unless the defender takes a set position, the path to the basket is the driving-man's, but he
cannot bowl over people en-route without being called
for fouls. The secret to success here is to have control of
your body and know where you are going and where
you can't go.

Which brings us to the layup, which is not really one
shot, though there is a basic layup shot. At the top of a
drive, a Baylor would use a two-hand underhand shot to
scoop the ball up and over the rim and into the hoop. I
also use this shot sometimes. The defenders are looking
for you to get your hands up to shoot and it catches

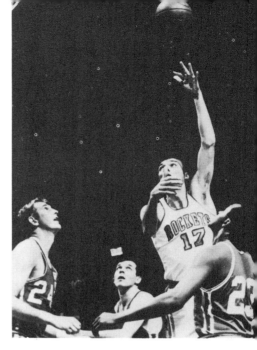

The hook shot as applied from head-on by
Henry Finkel (above) and from an awkward
angle by Bob Rule (below) under defensive
pressure. (San Diego Rockets and Seattle
SuperSonics)

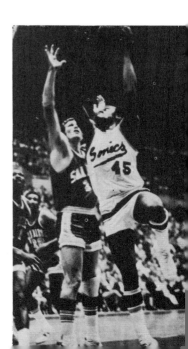

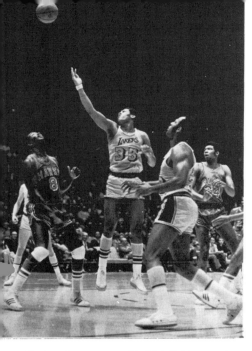

Rather than go up on big Walt Bellamy and risk a block, Rick Roberson lays one up underhand. (Photography, Inc.)

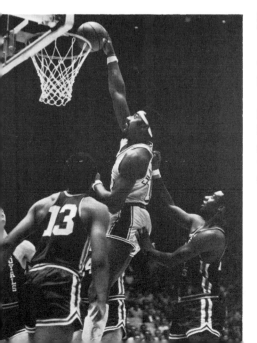

them unawares. As long as you have control of your body in the air, you have good control of the ball and can lift it up softly.

Some players seem to "hang" in the air, defying the laws of gravity. Well, for one thing, there is that moment of suspension at the peak of your jump. Secondly, the player who takes a driving leap at the basket, a sort of "broad-jump" or "long-jump," as it is now called, will be in the air longer, his momentum carrying him forward on a gradually curved leap, than the player who goes straight up. Often, as a driver takes off and moves through the air toward the basket, a defender in front of the basket will go up to attempt to block the shot. He will come down while the "long-jumper" remains in the air. Thus is the illusion of a player hanging suspended in space.

You must time your leap to reach the basket at the peak of your lift. At the conclusion of a short leap, a Wilt Chamberlain will stuff the ball down into the basket. He often does it with such force that he bangs his hand sore on the rim.

If you are tall enough and jump well enough to "stuff" the ball, by all means do it. Not because it is showy, but because it is the safest way to put the ball through the hoop. Of course, it is not legal on all levels. The colleges were the last to legislate against it, but it is perfectly permissible on the pro level. And fellows like Wilt, Reed, Elvin Hayes, Spencer Haywood, Connie Hawkins, and Mel Daniels are rather devastating in close to the hoop. Calvin Murphy, at 5-9, can also dunk the ball.

In the basic layup, you are driving on a dribble to the basket or running to the basket and taking a pass in the last stride. Preferably, drive to the basket from one side or the other instead of straight on. Approaching from the right side, jump up off your left foot while carrying the ball up in front of your body with both hands. As

Two views of Wilt Chamberlain's stuff-shot. Bottom left, he is seen from the side putting the ball over the rim as Tom Van Arsdale, Walt Wesley, and Oscar Robertson watch. Below, he is shown from overhead reaching to jam the ball home over Connie Hawkins and Paul Silas, while Jim Fox watches. (Photography, Inc.)

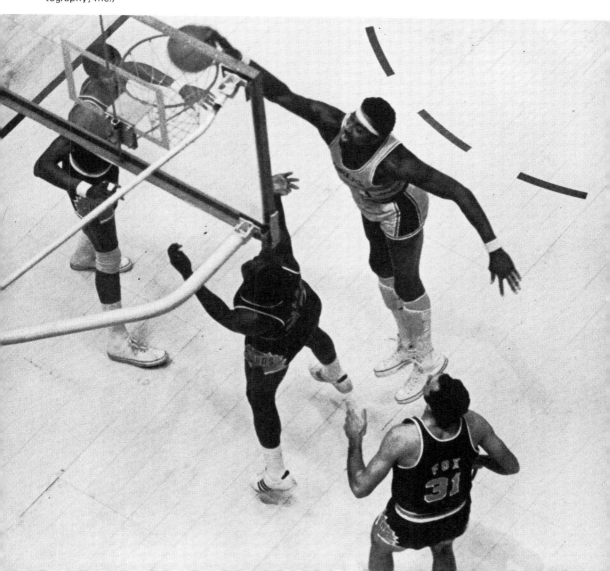

the ball clears the top of your head, drop your left hand off and extend the ball with your right hand to the backboard, placing it against the backboard about 6 inches above and to the right of the rim. Jump as high as you comfortably can, bringing your hand as close to the rim as you can, above it if you can. Practice will teach you where you have to place the ball to send it through the basket depending on your angle of approach. You do not have to and should not bang the ball off the backboard. Just place it there. Your momentum will do the rest.

It is really a difficult shot at first but will become the easiest shot later. It can be mastered with practice. Few put in the practice this shot deserves. It looks easy and they underestimate it. It is not easy to bank a ball home while driving and leaping at top speed with tremendous momentum, often against fierce defensive pressure. Yet fans are shocked when a pro blows one.

Take more of a high-jump than a long-jump. Learn where to take off from for your jump to put your hand right up to the spot on the backboard you are trying to reach. This is one of the few shots in which you use the backboard nowadays. In cramped quarters and positions underneath the board, it can be helpful to you. Carry the ball low and possibly even a bit behind you until you begin your jump, then hold your hand spread and behind and slightly beneath the ball as you go up to the board with it.

Normally you will take off on the opposite foot from the hand that is putting up the layup. The ball may be put up either with the hand under or behind the ball. The underhand method is softer, but the player may use either method and should work on both. He should work on going up with either foot, too, should circumstances force it. He must be able to lay the ball up left-handed from the left side, too. He must be able to layup the ball from anywhere with either hand. This takes practice.

An especially effective variation is the reverse layup. This is a valuable weapon when a tall defender is in position to block the player's layup attempt. It is a change-of-pace that throws the defenders off stride. Driving from the right the player keeps going beyond the basket to the other side, arrests his momentum, twists back, jumps up, and lays the ball up, usually with the opposite hand above and to the left of the bucket.

At first, this will be an awkward shot to master, but with practice you can get the timing down right. I found it a great help to me in the 1969 playoff finals against Boston and Bill Russell. I was able to get around him for a number of layups that he would have blocked if I had attempted them from the conventional side.

When attempting a layup straight-on, do not use the backboard, but lay it underhand as soft as possible just over the front rim. Be careful your momentum does not cause the ball to ricochet off the back rim. Preferably, if permissible and if possible for you, dunk the straight-on layups.

A most underrated form of shooting is the tap. The player's first concern is control of the ball. If he is not sure he can tap it back up successfully, he should grab it and come down with it, rebounding it, and then either go back for a close-in shot or pass the ball off. However, there are many situations where the tap is a good-percentage shot. If the ball comes off to you in the right place so you can tap it softly back to the basket, do it.

One of the problems with the tap is that it is misnamed. I am constantly surprised at how many experienced professionals try to tap the ball or bat wildly at it with their hands and fingertips. I don't know what it should be called, but I know how it should be done. The player should receive the ball in his spread hand, drawing the hand back to cushion the ball while bending his elbow, palming it or cupping it for a split second, then push it gently back up directly to the hoop, aiming to shove it softly just over the front rim of the hoop. With

A right-handed, backhanded reverse layup from the left side. This is in practice with Jim McMillian. I'm not sure I'd go this far in games. (Photography, Inc.)

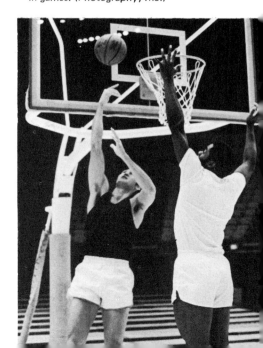

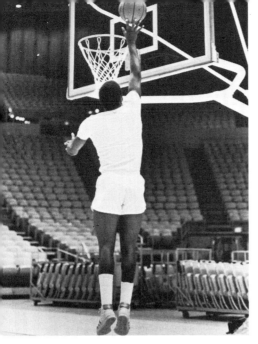

"Tapping," Jim McMillian has jumped, cushioned the ball in his palm, and is shoving it back up off his fingers as softly as possible in practice. (Photography, Inc.)

good body-control, this soft shot can be achieved even while the player is jumping.

The player can even practice this without a hoop, against any high wall. He can throw it up, then jump to palm the rebound and shove it back up softly to some spot on the wall. With practice, this can be a good-percentage shot. The centers will have the most chances for it, the guards the least, but the players who work on it may be surprised at how many opportunities to score this way develop in the course of a game for the aggressive, alert performer who goes to the hoop, who follows up shots, who is not shy about getting mixed up in the skirmishes under the basket.

There are many great shooters in the game today. In a classic sense, players could do worse than watch Jerry Lucas, Bob Love and John Havlicek shoot from the forward position, Kareem Jabbar, Bob Lanier, Willis Reed and Walt Bellamy shoot from the pivot or Oscar Robertson, Dave Bing, Walt Frazier, Gail Goodrich and myself shoot from the guard position. For pure shooting, it's hard to beat Flynn Robinson, Lucius Allen or Jon Mc-Glocklin. For more extreme styles, Connie Hawkins and Earl Monroe can be studied. For sheer scoring versatility, watch Rick Barry.

Elvin Hayes, Zelmo Beaty, Artis Gilmore, Julius Erving, Mel Daniels, Archie Clark, Charlie Scott, Ralph Simpson, Nate Archibald, Bill Bradley, John Brisker, Billy Cunningham, Larry Jones, Mack Calvin, Dave De-Busschere, Jim McDaniels, Larry Brown, John Brisker, Chet Walker, Willie Wise, Lou Hudson, Sidney Wicks, Jo Jo White, Glen Combs, Lou Dampier, George Lehmann and many others are around who have mastered the art of getting the ball in the hoop and should be studied.

As the game goes on, stretched rules make it harder and harder on scorers. What was designed as a noncontact game has become a bruising, crashing contest. Watch

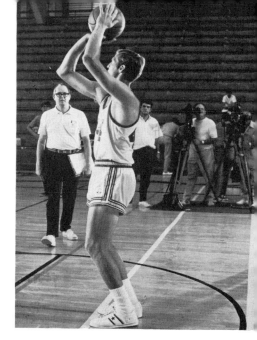

the way two tough centers push and pull each other
around in the pivot, jockeying for position, and you'll
see what I mean. It is incredible what these fellows can
do to each other without whistles being blown. When a
Wilt Chamberlain and a Willis Reed are healthy, they
give each other almost as much punishment in the pivot
as two heavyweight boxers in a ring. What you must
remember is that fellows such as Wilt and Willis are far
bigger, both taller and heavier, than the biggest heavy-
weights, even the Joe Fraziers and Muhammad Alis and
George Foremans.

A classic example of this is hand-guarding. Defenders
keep a hand or two hands on the players they are covering at all times, not only to keep track of where they are
and where they're going, but to shove them off stride as
much as possible. I am a victim of this, pushed and
pulled this way and that, but far from the only one. It is
hard to maintain my balance and quickness when being
pushed and pulled as though my defender were an octo-
pus. It's illegal in high school and college ball but permitted in pro ball. "No harm, no foul," they call it. No
harm, my foot. It drives me up the walls.

Watch the way a Dave Bing or a Rick Barry is man-
handled some time. Keep watching even when the tar-
geted player doesn't have the ball. Some of the defenders do everything but attack the big scorer with a stick.
It's something we have to adjust to. The best thing a
scorer can do to combat it is to keep moving, to make
the defender work to keep up with him. It takes a cool
head, finesse, and strength to resist it, and as I slow
down some I am beginning to be bothered by it.

You will draw fouls under this kind of defensing,
which brings us to perhaps the single most important
shot, the free-throw. I say "single most important" because the aggressive regular will draw a great many of
these in every game every season and he gets to shoot

Cameras turning, I practice free-throws for
instructional film for Sunkist Growers. Pub-
licist-producer Rene Henry is striding into
the picture. (William Eastabrook for Sunkist
Growers)

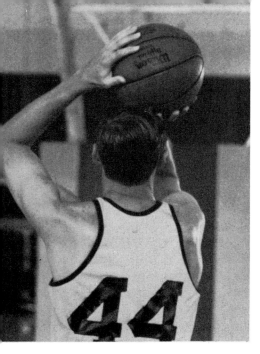

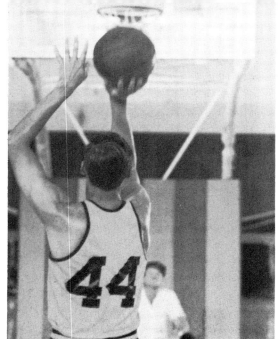

View from the rear of my free-throw technique: ball held in balance by my other hand until the last second, ball flat on my palm, limp-wrist follow-through. (William Eastabrook for Sunkist Growers)

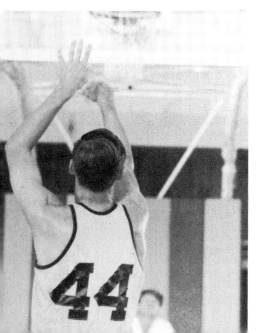

them standing still without defensive pressure. It is a sin the way some players throw these away. They are precious to the player individually and make the difference in the many games decided by a few points.

There is absolutely no reason why a player cannot approach perfection on free-throws. He should settle for no less than seven out of ten. Bunny Levitt, who went around giving exhibitions, once sank 499 in a row and 870 out of 871. Under the pressure of playing pro games, Bill Sharman once made 55 in a row during the regular season and 56 in a row during the playoffs. He won seven league free-throw titles and had the highest accuracy average ever for one season, 93 percent. His lifetime average was 88 percent.

Lifetime, I am in the top ten with 81 percent. My best single season was 87 percent, my longest streak was 31 in a row. I made more free-throws in one season, 840, and more in one playoff series, 137, than any other player. Usually, I will get one free-throw attempt to every two or three field attempts I take. This is a lot, and it's a shame when I waste them.

The one flaw in Wilt Chamberlain's fantastic statistical listing lies in free-throws. He has attempted more free-throws, more than 10,000, than any player ever, but has made only 51 percent of these. Four seasons he has been under 50 percent. One season he was around 44 percent. Oddly enough he holds the record with 28 of 32 in one game, but he has also missed more in one game, 22, more in one season, 578, and more in his career, more than 5,000, than any player ever.

In recent years it has become a mental block for Wilt. He has tried every conceivable style and was recently shooting from far back of the free-throw line and off to one side, banging the ball toward the backboard. The funny thing is, he makes them in practice. In games it is something else, and he is ridiculed for it. Wilt is a proud man with great records in his possession and possibly puts it down as unimportant.

Jabbar is around a 65-percent free-throw shooter, Reed around a 74-percenter. Among the best in basketball today are Flynn Robinson, Larry Siegfried, Oscar Robertson, Lou Hudson, Jack Marin, Gail Goodrich, John Havlicek, Rick Barry, Darell Carrier, Chet Walker, Mack Calvin, Louie Dampier, Bill Bradley, and Wally Jones. They all use slightly different styles, Barry even using the old underhand style. The important thing is to pick a style that feels comfortable to you and practice it, repeat it countless times, hundreds of times every week, until you groove it, then go on practicing it, keeping it in the groove. And when you get to the line in games, shut your mind to everything else except the mechanical motions you have mastered. Do it exactly the same way every time.

Use your best shot for your free shot. Not that I favor a jump shot, though a few do jump and are effective. But I am primarily a one-hand shooter, so I shoot one-hand free-throws. A good two-hand set-shooter should shoot two-hand free-throws. If a fellow is primarily an overhead shooter he can shoot his free-throws that way. The main thing, once you have practiced and grooved your free-throw, is to relax when you're at the line. Some players draw a deep breath. Others bounce the ball a few times. You're tired, maybe, and excited. Get calm before you shoot. You have ten seconds.

The one-hand free-throw is shot exactly as is the one-hand set shot. In the case of the free-throw, however, you're always standing in the same place, at the line, all alone with no defender facing up to you. The two-hand set-shot or overhead-shot free-throws are shot exactly the same as the basic shots from the field. I don't know anyone who ever took a hook-shot for a free-throw except Hot Rod Hundley, but he was clowning.

The one shot that is unique to the free-throw situation is the two-hand underhand shot. Spread your feet about shoulder-width or a little farther apart, in a comfortable position, toes even and on the line, body squared to the basket. Find a good balance. You may either hang your hands all the way down in a completely relaxed position or hold your hands at waist-level with your elbows slightly bent. Hold the ball in the balls of your palm and your fingertips on both sides and slightly on the underside of the ball with your fingers spread wide, but relaxed. Some players hold the ball on both sides but with their thumbs pointed at each other on the upper side of the ball. Find the grip you prefer.

Bend at the waist, cock your wrists, and bring the ball up by straightening your knees and swinging your arms forward. Release the ball with a slight snap of your wrists at about chest-level and continue on to a full follow-through that ends with your hands pointed at the basket. You do not have to shoot hard, just hard enough to loft the ball over that front rim. As the ball comes off your fingertips, a soft backspin will be imparted to it. Keep your head still, held up, eyes on the target at all times. Be aware of finding a groove and developing a rhythm.

Free-throws are about the only things that are given you in basketball, and even these you have to work for with aggressive play. Points are precious. It's a lot easier to sink two 1-point free-throws than one 2-point field-goal. Check the boxscores and see how many games are lost that could have been won with better free-throw shooting. Work at it and keep working at it. When you're given something in this game, don't give it away.

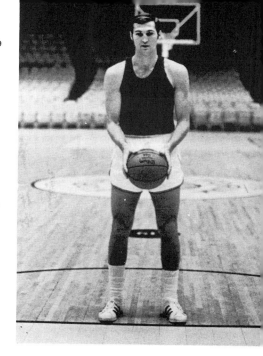

Two-hand, underhand free-throw form.
(Photography, Inc.)

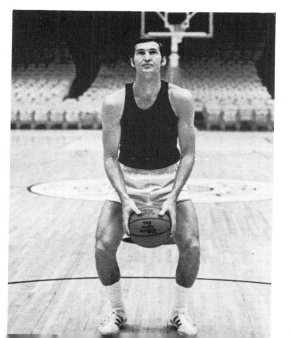

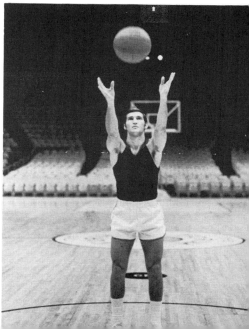

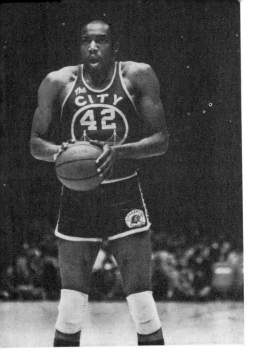

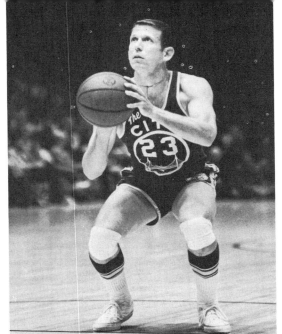

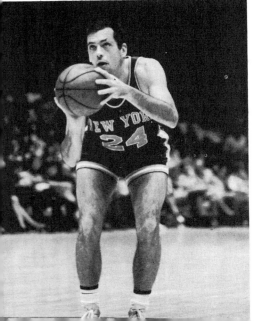

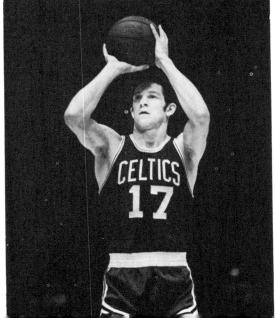

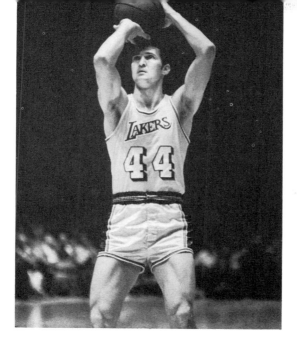

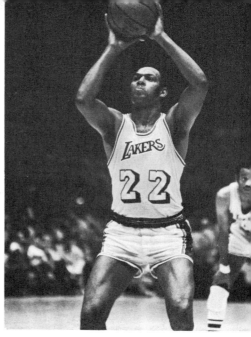

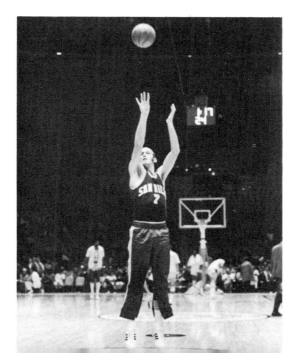

Varied free-throw styles: Facing page—upper left, Nate Thurmond drawing a relaxing deep breath; upper right, Jeff Mullins crouching and sighting; lower left, Bill Bradley, crouching more and sighting more intensely; lower right, John Havlicek, whose form is similar to mine. This page—upper left, "Zeke from Cabin Creek," a name I do not especially like; upper right, Elgin Baylor, who holds the ball quite high; lower left, Toby Kimball, who leaves his feet in a little jump as he shoots. (Photography, Inc.)

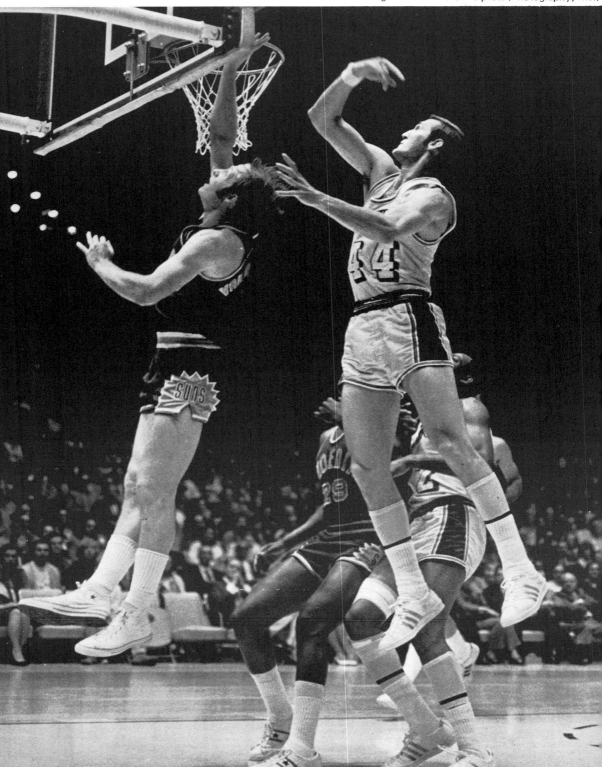

Even a little man can at times leap to block a shot. I'm 6-3 and here I'm up pretty high and have hooked a shot from Dick Van Arsdale off line. I'm sure it didn't discourage Dick, who with twin-brother Tom was an Indianapolis schoolboy and Indiana University star and is among the hardest-working and best all-around pros. (Photography, Inc.)

6. Defense and Rebounding

DEFENSE IS the single most important factor in the success or failure of a basketball team. I think more games are won on defense than on offense. The object of the game is to put the ball in the basket. But an equally important object is to stop a player from putting the ball in the hoop and it is harder to play defense than offense so those who master it succeed.

Most players and teams work more on offense than on defense. It's more fun. A boy can practice dribbling and shooting a great deal by himself, but he needs at least one other player and preferably a team to practice defense. And if he struggles to master defense, few of his friends and few fans will notice and he will not get much publicity and prestige from it. Even though everyone who ever played this game well knows that defense is as important as offense, only offense is considered in the selection of All-Star teams nine times out of ten.

The player is going to have to be unselfish, he is going to have to put the team first, in order to develop his defensive play. Because of the emphasis on offense from the time a player starts practicing and then plays in

One of the smoothest and surest defensive players and ballhawks in basketball, Walt Frazier slides past the screen I am putting on Mike Riordan to keep up with a dribbling Johnny Egan, who is one of the many small men who've succeeded in the sport. (Photography, Inc.)

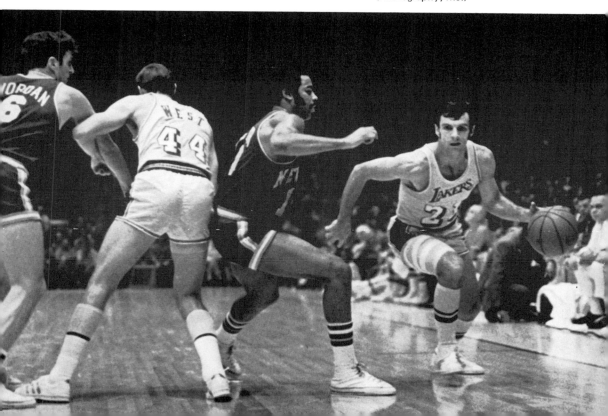

games, good shooters are a dime a dozen while good defenders are rare. I have seen many fine shooters come into pro ball who failed to become stars and often failed to make teams because they were not good all-around players and often because they didn't play defense. A player who is not a great shooter can make a place for himself with great defensive play.

I won't lie to you that it's a magic door to success. Many coaches, perhaps most coaches, lean toward offense and don't give fine defensive players the credit they deserve and a place among the starters. But many do. Within the fraternity of basketball people the great defender is more respected than are most great shooters. A player should take personal pride in his defense even if he doesn't have public recognition. It's only in the last few years of my career that my defensive abilities were recognized, yet I honestly believe I am a better defensive than an offensive player and am prouder of my defense than of my offense.

I am not just saying this for effect. I mean it sincerely. I don't always get to use my defensive abilities to their fullest. Because I am a top scorer I seldom am used to defend the other team's best offensive guards due to the fear I'll wear myself out or foul out. However, when not paired with a good defensive guard I am often put on a top player on the other team and I take pride in doing a job on him. What kind of job can I do? I can force him out of his favorite spots on the court, take his best shots and passes away from him, and steal the ball from him a fair number of times. These won't show in the stats, but they're as important as points.

My main assets in my defense are my quickness, my long arms for my height, and my anticipation. My long arms are a freak of nature. And as long as players oppose me they never seem to realize what a great reach I have, and this enables me to get my hands on the ball when it is least expected. The anticipation comes from experience, having observed closely the players I've played,

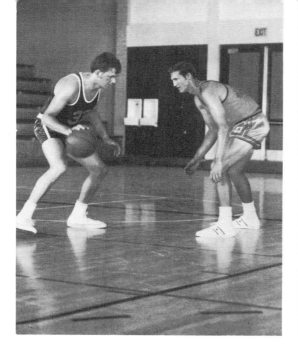

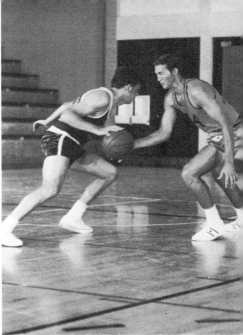

and from concentration. I pay more attention to defense than most players. If I'm tired, I'm more inclined to rest on offense than on defense. I think all players should. It's a lot easier to play four-man offense than it is to play four-man defense.

My handicap on defense is my lack of height, even with my long arms and quickness. While my 6-3 is an adequate height for guards, a lot of 6-5 and 6-6 guards are coming to the top these days, and it's tough to give away these inches to good jumpers. And it's very difficult for me to switch to guarding forwards, who seldom are under 6-5 and are often 6-7 and 6-8, and impossible for me to guard the 6-10, 6-11, 7-foot centers. Also, it's very hard for me to get rebounds away from the big men up front who dominate the boards.

Since defense essentially is the art of getting the ball from the offense, I include rebounding in this part of the game. There is offensive rebounding as well as defensive rebounding, of course, but essentially both are concerned with getting the ball back after you've given it up, if only through having taken a shot. It is because of blocking shots and serving as the last line of defense

Here in practice I move to my left to lure Rod Hundley into going into a drive on my right, but then lean back, reach out a hand, and take the ball right off his dribble. He might have made it past me had he shifted his dribble to his left hand. (William Easta-brook for Sunkist Growers)

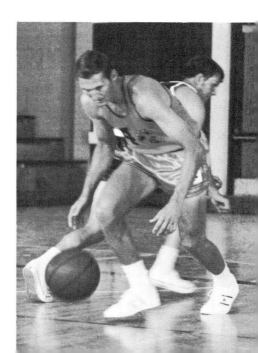

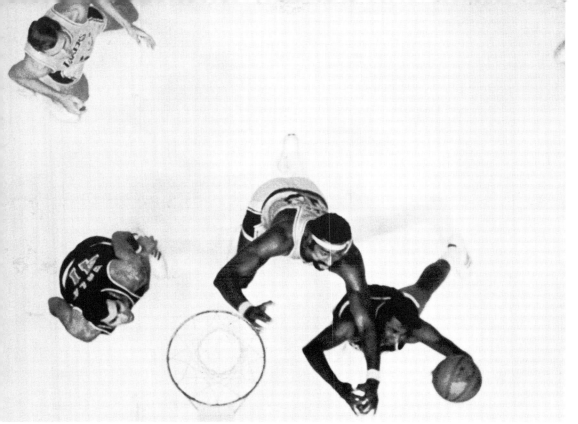

From overhead, Jerry Chambers, although being punished as Wilt reaches in, takes a rebound away from Chamberlain with Neal Walk and me watching. (Photography, Inc.)

under the basket and because of their rebounding that the big centers dominate this game the way a guard, no matter how individually excellent, ever could.

If I were a much better player than a Bill Russell or a Jabbar, and I am not, I still could not be as valuable to my team as they have been to their teams for the simple reason that they can get the ball for their teams and thus dominate the games as I never could. It is not their scoring that makes them dominant, but their all-around play, especially their defense and rebounding. Kareem is a super-scorer, Russell was not, but both have dominated this game. The offense is a plus, but it is the defense that means the most. Wilt's defense and rebounding meant more to us in 1972 than his greatest scoring years meant to his teams. He was truly a dominant force.

Yes, my value is doubled by my defense, by the balls I get with steals and the baskets I prevent with guarding. I've said no defensive player can stop a top scorer and I stick to that. I don't think any defensive player can stop me, no more than I or any other defender can stop an Oscar Robertson, or a Kareem Abdul-Jabbar. What I can do, what any defensive player can do, is to make it harder for them to control the ball, make good plays, and get good shots. To repeat: Take just a few baskets away from me or any other offensive player and you may have decided the game. It is a game of percentages. Ordinarily, certain players will wind up with certain totals. Change these and you change the course of the game.

There have been some superb defensive players in basketball. I think K. C. Jones is about the best I ever observed at guard.

I think the best team I've seen in the NBA was the Boston Celtics of 1963-64, the year after Cousy retired, because it was the most aggressive defensive team I've ever known. K. C. moved in as a regular. Bill Russell, the game's single most devastating defensive force ever, remained a regular. Red Auerbach coached defense and everyone on that team played aggressive defense. This team had no great offensive edge on its foes. Some teams scored almost as much or even more. But no other team took the ball away as this one did.

There have been many other great defensive players in my time in pro ball. Among guards, Lenny Wilkens, Walt Frazier, Jerry Sloan, Joe Caldwell, and Dick Van Arsdale stand out in my mind; among forwards, Bill Bridges, Gus Johnson, Dave DeBusschere, Rudy La-Russo, Tom Sanders, and Tom Van Arsdale; among centers, Jabbar, Nate Thurmond, Willis Reed, Wes Unseld, Zelmo Beaty, and Wilt Chamberlain. As I write this, Milwaukee, New York, and Chicago are outstanding on defense. Thus it's no surprise that they are among the best teams.

Defense should be the most consistent part of a player's game. He should not go in streaks the way a player may do on offense. His job may be tougher from game to game depending on whom he's facing, but he should

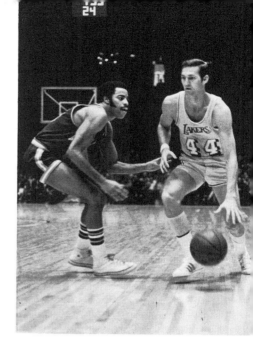

Here I am watched intently by defensive specialist Walt Frazier, who soared to stardom from Southern Illinois University. (Photography, Inc.)

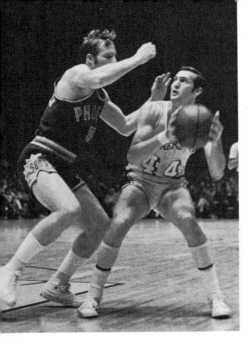
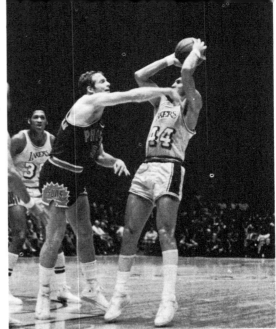

I haven't faced many defenders in the NBA better than these. In the top two pictures, Dick Van Arsdale, who I feel is about the toughest defender around these days, applies his usual relentless, physical style on me. When I get in close, bigger forwards often pick me up. At the lower left, former teammate Rudy LaRusso, a hardworking defensive cornerman, goes up with me; at the lower right, one of the stronger defenders, Gus Johnson, keeps me company. (Photography, Inc.)

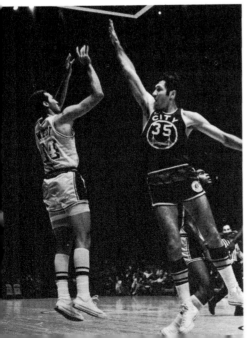
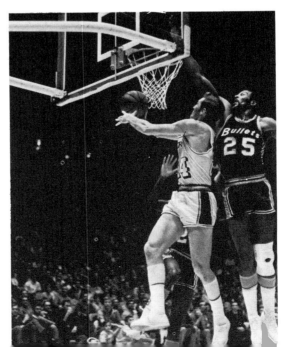

be able to do the same sort of job every time. Defense should be a constant, stabilizing factor.

On defense the player must hustle at all times. The free ball is yours, so go after it. I think the most over-looked aspect of Boston's run of eleven titles in thirteen seasons was its ability to come up with loose balls. No matter how much the Celtics won, they outhustled teams that should have been hungrier. Convert these into three or four baskets a game and you have the difference between winning and losing, especially in critical games.

As a coach, Bill Sharman stresses details. He learned this from his years with the Celtics, studying the action and observing that almost invariably there were key games that were won by a last shot or in overtime. He says details provided the difference, and I agree with him.

You have to put a lot into the game. Not "110 per-cent," a phrase that makes me sick. No one can give 110 percent. No one has more than 100 percent in him. But you can give everything you've got, which is 100 per-cent. Few of us ever even approach 100 percent. Think about it. For full games, are you giving 50 per-cent? Or 60 percent? Or 70 percent? Strive for 100 per-cent and you may give 80 or 90 percent, and that's a lot.

It's on defense that this is most necessary, because defense is mastery of fundamentals, complete concentra-tion, and hard work. You are going to have to learn as much about your opponents as you can. The offensive player has that built-in edge. He knows what, when, and where he's going to do his thing. When he moves, there's going to be a split-second before the quickest player can react. Cut down this edge by observing your foes.

If you know that a player always shoots when he gets the ball in a certain position you can anticipate this and move with him. If you know one always passes from certain places on the court, anticipate it and get in posi-tion to prevent or hamper it. Generally, try to force him

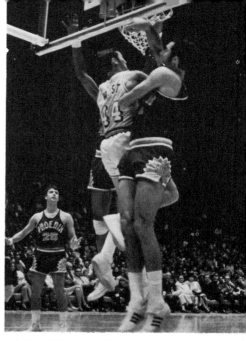

A Jerry West sandwich is formed by de-fenders Connie Hawkins (on my far side) and Jim Fox. At 6-3, I may be forcing my shot from under the hoop against the 6-8 Hawkins and 6-10 Fox. It does get rough in there sometimes. (Photography, Inc.)

Here I give some defensive instruction to son Mark guarding dribbling son Michael. He is close enough to be called for a foul but he may have his kid brother cornered and I forgot my whistle. (Photography, Inc.)

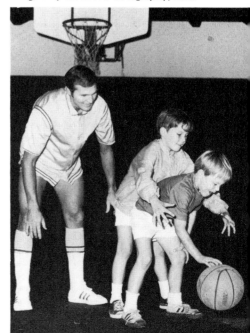

outside, away from the basket, into corners. Specifically, try to force him away from his favorite places on the court. If he's a much better driver than he is an outside shooter, play him loose. If vice versa, play him tight.

Don't overdo this. As much as possible, don't commit yourself before he does. He is trying to draw you into this. Learn his fakes so you can better resist them. Don't take false tips. Be sure of yourself before you overplay an opponent. Nothing is 100 percent, but play the percentages. If a fellow seldom hits a jump-shot from beyond 15 feet, let him have these so you can take better shots away from him, but don't get discouraged if he hits one or two. Guard the man, not the ball. Of course, you guard him when he doesn't have the ball, too. But what you are doing then is trying to prevent the ball from getting to him in his favored places.

Learn your assignment in each of many different defensive patterns your team uses. Man-to-man is the most popular defense in basketball and the only one permissible in pro ball, although the rules are stretched into subtle variations of zone defenses. For example, the big center who never wanders far from the basket on defense no matter where his opponent goes is playing a one-man zone. In a zone the players guard areas of the court instead of opponents. It is used to some extent in high school and college ball and adds variety to the game. I see no reason why it should be barred from pro ball, although I do not favor it.

During the 1970-71 season, Joe Mullaney, then my coach on the Lakers, took advantage of NBA rules against the zone to isolate me on one side of the court. Thus I could not be double-teamed. No one else could help out my guard. And, frankly, it is very hard for any single player to guard me one-on-one. This was done when the Lakers had a lot of injuries, and I was asked to carry more of an offensive load than usual. And it was successful to some extent, although our opponents screamed bloody murder. However, I didn't like it much more than they did. It was exhausting, and I prefer to be part of the team, looking for the pass as well as the shot.

There are many kinds of zones. There's a two-one-two, in which two men play up front, one in the middle, and two in back. The middleman becomes a rover, free to help out. There's a two-three, which is good against an imposing pivot, since it puts three men near the basket. There's a three-two, which is good for teams that like to fast-break, because it puts three men near midcourt in good position to go the second their team gets the ball. And there's the two-two-one, which most pro teams mesh into their man-to-man. There are other kinds. There are kinds of man-to-man defenses, including those that stress pressing, double-teaming, or switching. The important thing is to learn your assignment in each.

In the zone you have a specific territory to cover. In the man-to-man you have a man to cover. Make sure you know who he is at all times. This may sound easy but substitutions complicate it. It is not unusual for two men to wind up covering the same man while another goes unguarded. By the time you discover this you've probably given up some precious points.

The key thing is to stay between your man and the basket. The second key is to stay between your man and the man he wants to get the ball to. The defender's first job is to cover his man; his second is to cover up for his teammates.

When an offensive player gets between you and the man you are guarding he is setting up a block, or a screen, sometimes called a "pick," to enable his teammate to drive around you or shoot free from you. You may go around the screen, provided you feel you have time to pick up your man again before he has done his thing. You may try to fight through the screen at the risk of committing a foul. Or you may switch, hollering to the nearest teammate to pick up your man, in which case you must pick up your teammate's man.

As on offense, you will have to make decisions swift-

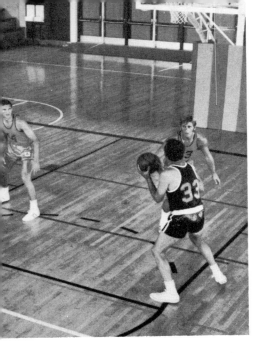
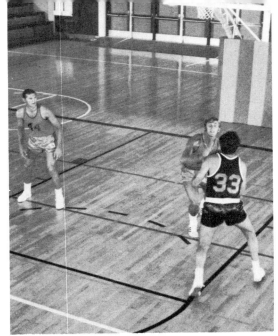

Here's an example of successful switching in practice. I'm guarding Art Williams and Pat Riley is guarding Rod Hundley, with the ball. Rod fakes a shot, causing Pat to jump up. While Pat's in the air, Rod drives around him for the basket. Seeing this, I leave my man to pick Rod up and get there in time to block his layup attempt. (William Eastabrook for Sunkist Growers)

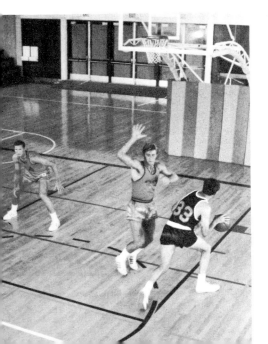
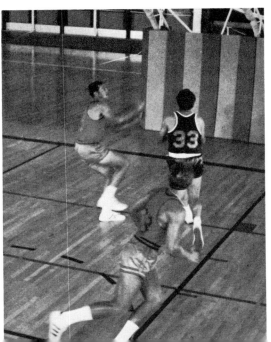

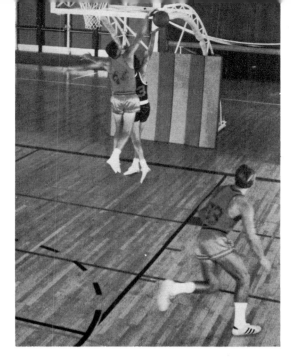

ly as play develops, so experience will improve you as you go along. If you see a free foe on the way to the basket you have to cover him, but if it causes you to free your man to be in a better position than the original player, you should not go toward him. You will make mistakes, but you have to keep working, hustling and developing good judgment from having been in this position many times before. Generally speaking, a switching defense is the best. It puts the whole team into defense and provides for coverage of all foes. However, smart offensive teams will use your switches to mismatch you against perhaps a taller or quicker player, so it is not without its problems.

Within the framework of any man-to-man defense there are certain targets to aim at. You try to minimize the other team's strengths and maximize its weaknesses. You try to press the fellow who has the ball who does not handle the ball well. You try to force the other team to give him the ball. You try to stop the best shooter from getting the ball, especially in the places from which

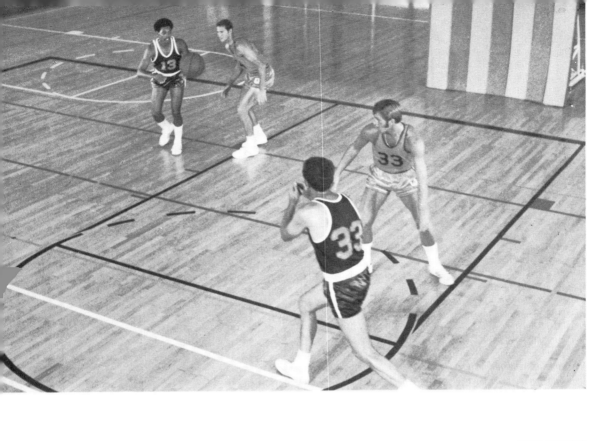
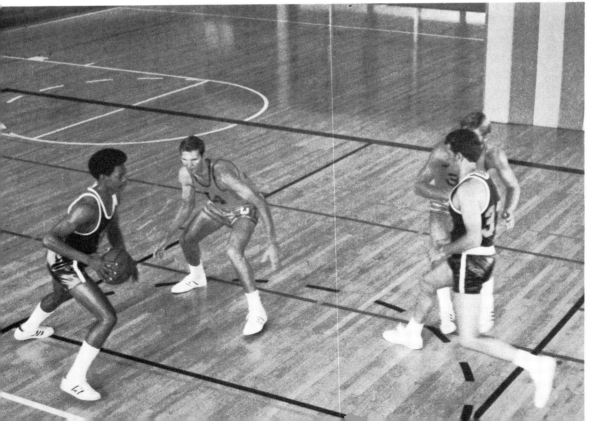

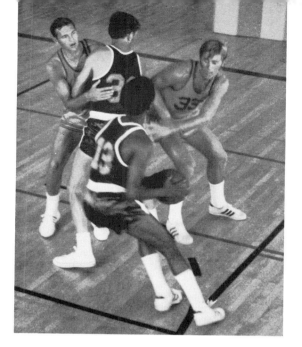 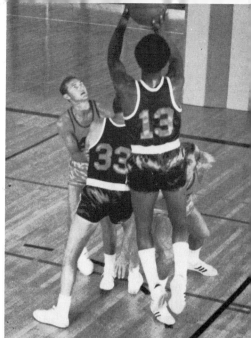

he shoots it best. You try to force the offensive team outside, as far from the basket as possible, or you can collapse your defensive strength in the middle and try to lure your foes into this congested zone. You are especially careful with the other team's key men.

You do these things with variations of overplaying. If a man goes right much better than left, you play him to the right. Or if his best play is to the left, you play more to the left. Often you will overplay a man inside to force him to go outside. If he is not a good dribbler or is a slow passer, you may wish to gamble more than usual by going for steals, but resist the temptation to commit yourself too much or lunge too often, taking yourself out of the play. To steal the ball you have to go after it, but recognize the risk you are taking. Sometimes, blocking or deflecting a pass is as valuable as a steal. Anything that breaks up the other team's play is helpful.

It often helps to double-team certain men. If there are players who are so good they require extra guarding or players who are vulnerable, you can benefit by working on them. Two men can force a good shooter to give up on getting off a shot and pass the ball to someone less

On these two pages, here's a screen that beats me on defense. Again, I'm guarding Art Williams and Pat Riley is guarding Rod Hundley, with the ball. Rod passes to Art and puts a pick on Pat. Art dribbles so tightly on Rod I wind up on the other side of him, blocked out with Pat, as Art goes up for an open shot. (William Eastabrook for Sunkist Growers)

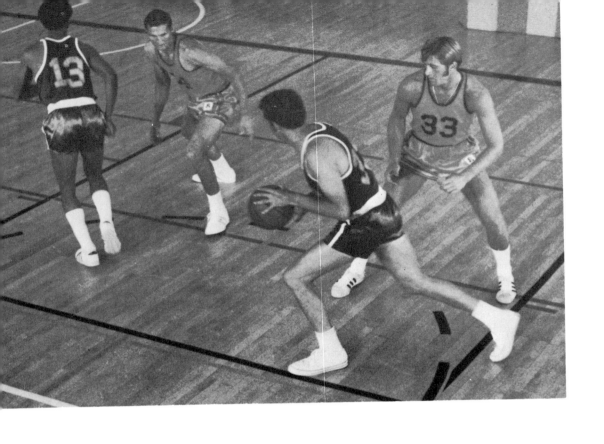

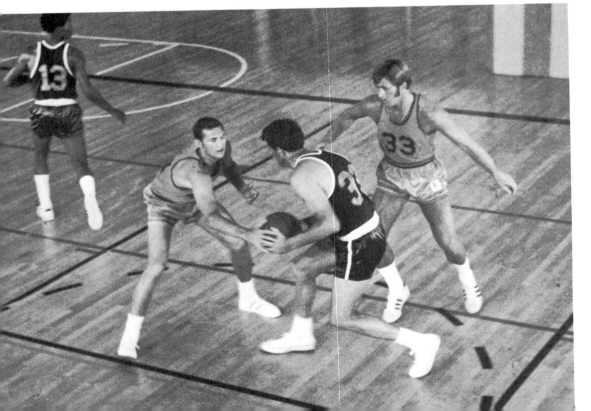

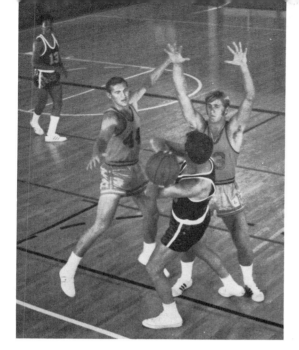

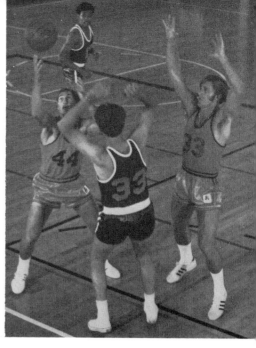

On these two pages, a double-team pays off in practice. I'm guarding Art Williams and Pat Riley is on Rod Hundley. As Rod dribbles to his left, I leave my man to join Pat on him and we exert sufficient pressure to cause him to give up on his dribble and attempt a desperate off-balance pass, which I can block and pick off. Remember, the defenders can't touch you or they'll foul. If the pressure is too much for the ballhandler, he should call a time-out. (William Eastabrook for Sunkist Growers)

dangerous. In these cases you drop off your man to lend a hand on a teammate guarding the man with the ball. But you must always remember that you are leaving your man, thus it is dangerous. And you must always be prepared to return to him swiftly.

Sometimes it is helpful to apply extra pressure to the entire opposing team. You may put on a pressing defense all over the court or only after the offensive team has moved across midcourt. In a pressing defense you play closer to the offensive players than usual; in a sense, you are all over them. Usually, you are going after the ball with your hands, but it is possible to press merely with aggressive use of your body without using your hands at all. There are many benefits to the press. You will force foes into errors and get many steals, deflections, and loose balls. You will force them to make hurried moves, you will disconcert them. This pressing style is especially effective on the lower levels, against teams that are inexperienced. And if you are a running team you will pick up many fast-breaks on your foes.

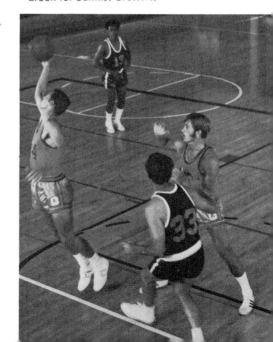

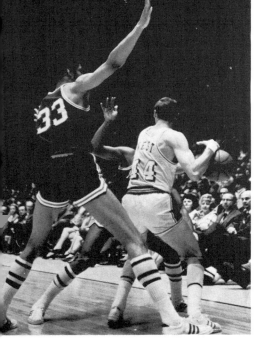

I'm hemmed in by a double-team put on by towering Jabbar and Oscar Robertson. (Photography, Inc.)

Applying an all-court press, the guards, Pat Riley and myself, pick up Art Williams and the dribbling Rod Hundley. Fast passing is the best way to disrupt a press, which is effective but exhausting and risky. (William Eastabrook for Sunkist Growers)

However, there are also problems and risks. It is exhausting to press a lot and dangerous if you are not in the best possible condition. If you are slow you can't press effectively. If the other team handles the ball well it will exploit your overplaying and will move the ball quickly around you, or it will wind up with many one-man breakaways, or two-on-one or three-on-one breaks.

Pressing is not a cautious defense. But against the right team, or when you need the ball badly, it can be a tremendous tactic. Pressing has worked well at times in the NBA, as the offensive team must cross the midcourt line within 10 seconds and has only 24 seconds in which to get off a shot. On other levels there is more time.

The most important part of your posture in playing defense is your balance. The offensive player is trying to throw you off-balance, so you must strive to maintain it at all times and be able to go in any direction quickly. He has that edge on you, and when he makes a move you must react as swiftly as possible. Get down fairly low. Bend at the knees. Bend forward from the waist. Spread your feet comfortably. Keep your weight slightly

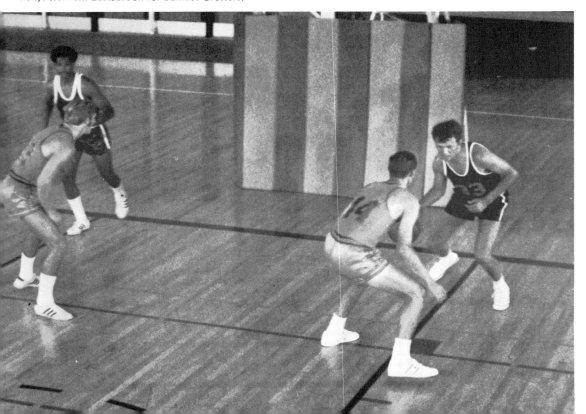

forward so that you are not flat-footed. Keep one hand
high and one low and both slightly out to cover as much
up-and-down and side-to-side area as possible. Keep
switching your high hand and your low hand. Keep moving them, but don't wave them wildly. Move one hand
with the ball at all times. Keep one hand in front of the
shooter's face to obscure his vision. Don't ever drop
your hands completely. Don't ever give him a free path
for a pass or a shot.

Unless deliberately pressing, stay 2 to 3 feet away
from him. He may start a drive, but you'll be able to
react before he is past you. As you sense or see that he is
going to pass or shoot, move up on him but resist his
fakes. Try not to lunge or jump, which will make you
vulnerable to his drive. As you move to cover him, shuffle, never cross your feet. Crossing your feet restricts
your mobility and throws you off-balance. Learn to
shuffle, side-to-side and front-to-back, right foot toward
left foot, left foot away, right foot toward left foot, and
so forth.

Keep your feet spread far apart. Usually, your feet
are squared on your foe, but if you want to overplay
him in one direction or the other you can stagger your
stance by placing one foot forward in that direction.
Keep stealing glances at your man's belt-buckle. He may
fake you out with movements of his eyes, head, shoulders, or feet, but he will not be going anywhere until his
gut goes there.

Your defensive tactics are similar whether your man
has the ball or not. Even if he does not have the ball you
should try to stay close to him, keep track of him, be in
a position to defend when he gets the ball. In many cases
you will try to keep him from getting the ball. In some
cases you may try to do this by "fronting him." This is
done a lot in the pivot, where the big man may be impossible to contain once he gets the ball. However, fronting foes is risky, because if he gets the ball he is behind

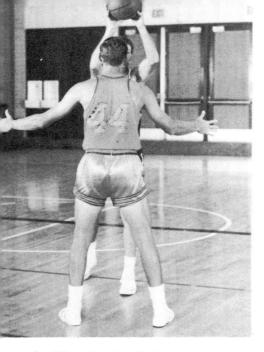
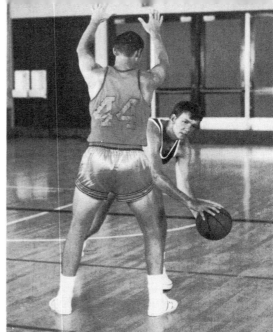

In all these, I apply defensive pressure on
Rod Hundley. In the first two, I do not
move properly, presenting him with a clear
path to a pass. In the others, I stay with
him, going where he goes. (William Eastabrook for Sunkist Growers)

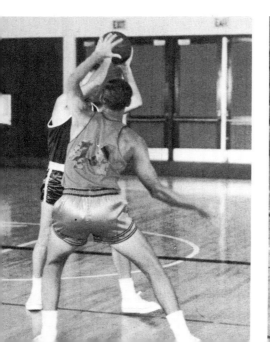
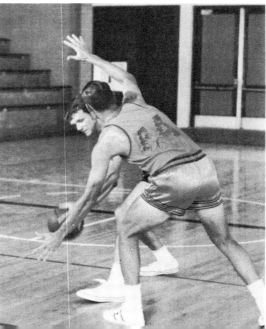

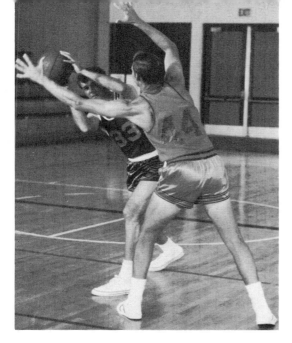
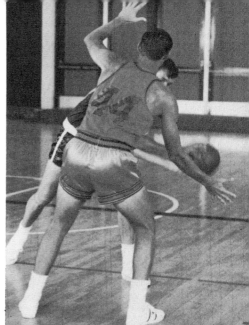

you, on his way to the basket. Usually, it is best to play behind the man, between him and the basket.

Start with a short step to get going quickly. Practice to develop a swift, sure shuffle. If your foe is getting past you, make a quick pivot in his direction, wheeling to get your head, shoulder, and arm thrusting in that direction, make a short sprint, then stop by planting your lead foot firmly, drop your hips low and bend at the knees to resume a low center of gravity, then regain your balance as quickly as possible. Generally, you can run faster than he can dribble, so you will be able to catch up to him most times. Never turn your back on him.

When outnumbered, when you are the lone man back with two offensive players coming at you, you can't cover both perfectly, so don't try to steal the ball. Play the angles on them. Stay between them. Fake a move at them and retreat. Fake and retreat. Think of yourself as the pointed part of a triangle. Stay equidistant between them and stay between them and the basket. Fake and retreat. Make them work as hard as possible. They have to handle the ball. One mistake and their advantage is

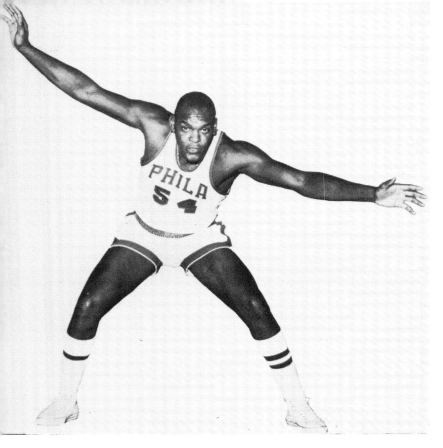

Luke Jackson, at 6-9 and 240, assumes defensive position. Are you ready to get the ball or yourself past him? (Philadelphia 76ers)

lost. Most times they'll beat you. But if you work at it, making them work at it, you'll upset them more times than they expect.

When you are on defense one-on-one, always be alert for the possibility of stealing the ball, of batting it out of his hands or off his dribble or off his pass. As much as possible, reach for the ball with your arm and hand, don't lunge for it with your whole body. If you miss it on a lunge, you've lost your man. Lunge only when you are sure you can get to the ball and go with it.

Look for the pattern of his dribble and his moves. Watch for those times he waves the ball around or holds it loosely in front of him or has only one hand on it. Try to stay on your toes, in balance, and within reach of him at all times. When you see the ball exposed, reach swiftly for it without diving at it. Trying to go around you, he may be vulnerable to a steal. Sometimes you, even though the defender, can fake him by threatening a steal attempt in one direction, then suddenly reaching out in the other. You can reach the ball as well with your left hand as with your right.

I should say here that I am an unorthodox defensive player. The player must find what works and what does not work for him. When Bill van Breda Kolff first came to coach the Lakers he thought I did certain things "wrong." But as he saw they went right for me, he changed his mind. For example, I will often deliberately open myself up for a player to drive around me on one side, tempting him to drive around me, because I know I can reach over and steal the ball from him as he goes past me. This is dangerous and I don't preach it as a thing to practice. I can do it because of my unusual quickness and long arms. This quickness enables me to "cheat" to one side or the other. I also have a Chamberlain in the middle to back me up. But if you don't have physical talents along these lines, and a great defensive man behind you, play a more conservative, more careful defensive game based on the best fundamentals.

Make as few mistakes as possible on defense. If you make a mistake, do what you can to make up for it. If you lose your man, pick up someone else's. Go with the flow of play as much as possible. Roll inside to provide added protection around the basket.

As soon as your man shoots, wheel around and get between him and the basket, thrusting your back at him, blocking him off from the rebound. Do this as soon as any man shoots. Look for the rebound or the loose ball that comes out of a scramble. Talk to your teammates to keep them aware of what's happening to you. If you lose

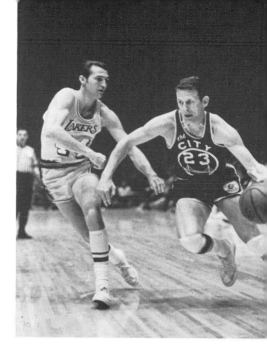

Losing my man, I fail to keep up with Jeff Mullins on a dribble-drive. I have crossed my legs, he has gotten away, so I can only hope someone else picks him up. (Photography, Inc.)

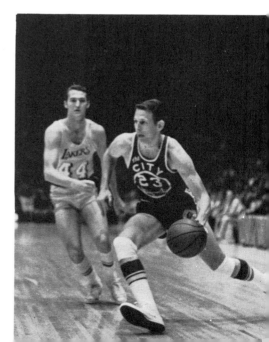

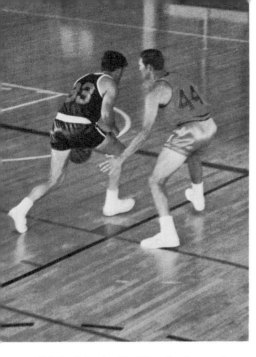
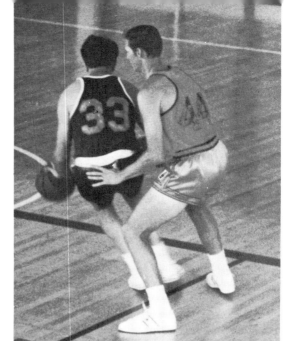

Tightly defensing Rod Hundley in practice,
I force him to reverse and force a hook. Rod
has been known to force shots before, but it
is amazing how I handle the old guy. (William Eastabrook for Sunkist Growers)

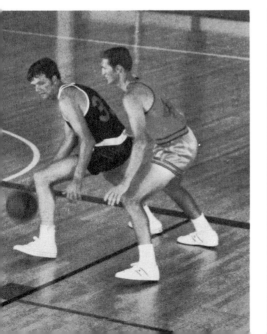
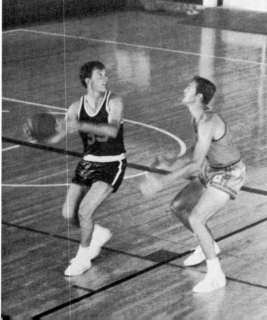

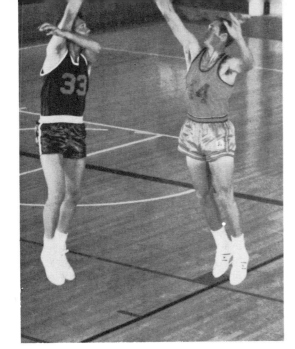

your man, yell it out. If you're going to switch, yell it out. The man inside the switch should call for it, because he sees the screen developing in front of him and can help his teammate by taking his man instantly.

Each position makes special defensive demands on a player. The guard works the hardest on defense, as he defends the opponent's guards, who usually bring the ball upcourt. The guard must be ready to fall back on defense at all times and is usually the first man back. He can't just rush in to join the offensive scramble after a shot by a teammate. And when the guard drives to the basket, he must be prepared to get back into defensive position as quickly as possible. The guard usually defends the quickest and most agile players in the most wide-open territory.

On the other hand, the guard is usually farthest from the basket and so less vulnerable to being scored on. The forward must guard the cornerman, who is close enough to the basket to shoot, who can drive for the bucket, who can feed the pivot a pass that will result in a score. The defender must compromise, staying close enough to the cornerman to impede a shot and far enough away to

Wilt Chamberlain goes high to attempt to block a jumping hook by Elvin Hayes. (Photography, Inc.)

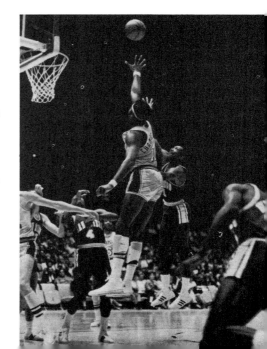

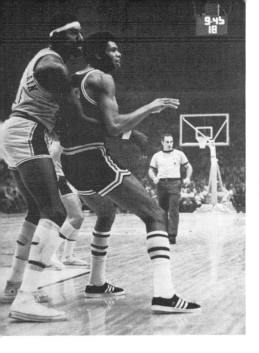

protect against a drive. The defensive forward must keep his hands up high to protect against the overhead shot and the looping pass to the pivot.

The defensive center has great responsibility, as he is the last line of defense. As pioneered by Bill Russell, shot-blocking has become one of the dominant defensive tactics in the sport. The expert shot-blocker accomplishes a number of things. First of all, of course, he blocks the shot itself. Then he discourages the shooter. He embarrasses him, though it is becoming commonplace. If it is done to him enough, the shooter will begin to rush his shot or put on an unnatural arc, which usually ruins it. And the shot-blocker discourages entire teams, causing them to stop driving into his territory, taking away the inside game from them, and forcing them outside. Stats aren't kept on blocked shots, but with them Bill Russell, Wilt Chamberlain, and Kareem Abdul-Jabbar have become dominant players who frustrate foes and force them from their normal styles.

It is not easy to block shots. The shooter gets the jump on the defender, who must react swiftly and take advantage of that moment at the top of a jump-shot when a player "hangs" to bat the ball back down his throat. It takes precise timing, which must be perfected with practice. And there is an extreme risk of fouling. But it is a wonderful weapon that players should use more, especially noncenters. For example, there is no reason guards can't block more shots from guards of similar size. The low shot and the flat shot are most vulnerable to being blocked.

The defensive center has more immediate responsibilities, too. He is more concerned about keeping the ball from the offensive center than about stopping the offensive center once he gets the ball. Frankly, on the pro level, it is very hard for the defensive center to stop the offensive center when he gets the ball in close. It is difficult for a Wilt Chamberlain to stop a Kareem Abdul-Jabbar and vice versa. The 7-footer is just too close to

Two aspects of the battle of the super-centers are shown here in classic camera work by Wen Roberts. Above, leaning on one another and virtually embracing, Wilt Chamberlain and Jabbar await a pass. Below, Wilt tries to shoot while Bill Russell goes to block. (Photography, Inc.)

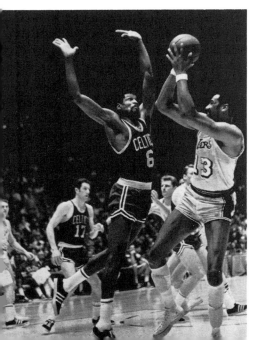

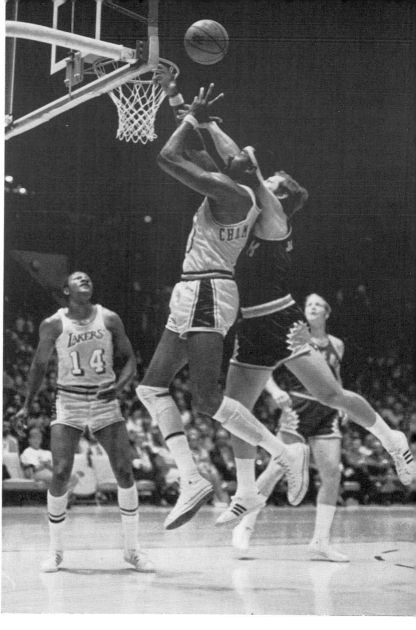

Banging into Big Wilt, a defender jars and ruins his layup attempt. (Photography, Inc.)

the bucket to be stopped very often. So more than any other player the defensive center will often front his man, or semifront him by playing to his side—on whatever side the ball is on—reaching in front of him with a waving hand to discourage the passer.

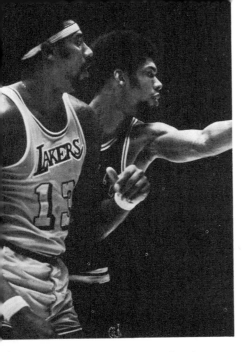

Defending Wilt, "siding" him rather than fronting him, Kareem pokes an arm out as he strives to prevent the pass from ever reaching his opposing pivot. (Photography, Inc.)

Having lost me, Bob Lewis reaches in desperately and fouls me. (Photography, Inc.)

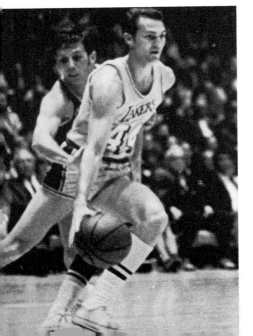

Basically, once the offensive center has the ball the defensive center moves to stay between him and the basket. With his body he tries to force him as far away as possible. That's why there is a tremendous amount of bumping and shoving by the centers in close to the hoop. There are two big men fighting for territorial advantages in precious areas near the basket. You bump and shove and hand-guard as much as is permitted to gain as much advantage as you can while trying not to foul out of games and give free-throws that can cost you games.

There are players who foul out repeatedly. You should play only as aggressively as the ref and your own body-control permit. In anything you do, you should get to know your limits and never exceed them. Attempting to do what you have not learned to do well can only cause you grief. If you do get in foul trouble, play your own game. Don't get overly cautious, because this is like handing your man a tremendous advantage. Don't play beyond yourself and don't play beneath yourself.

If a player beats you, he beats you. Let it go. Try to get him next time. Most often, fouls are committed by frustrated players who have lost their men and are trying to get even by playing overaggressively. Don't throw away your limit of fouls and don't give away free-throws. Make them earn their baskets. Play with as much aggressiveness as your ability permits and you will commit only the most unavoidable fouls.

Be aware of the capabilities of your opponents. For example, the lower the level on which you are playing, the less dangerous the center may be. On the high school level and lower, many tall but awkward and mediocre players are in the pivot. The defensive center does not have to risk fronting them, because he can stop them defensively. Suit the style you use to the abilities of your opponents.

Two ways you can get the ball from your foes is with jump-balls and rebounding. There are some jump-balls in every game, and the player should not dismiss them as sheer chance situations. If you are right-handed, stand with your right shoulder angled at the path the ball will take with your right foot angled to the imaginary line between you and your foe. Keep your legs comfortably spaced. Too wide a stance will weigh against the height of your jump. Hold your arms in comfortably close to

Why are all these Cleveland Cavaliers standing around while Wilt goes up? Answer that and you may also learn why Cleveland had such troubles in its first season. (Photography, Inc.)

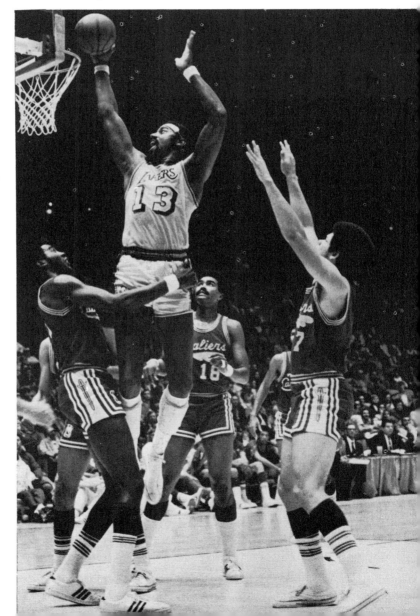

your body with your elbows bent. Hold your right hand head-high. Crouch into a coiled but balanced position.

As the official throws the ball up the player coils a bit tighter, then pushes upward from the knees and feet, thrusting up and reaching as far as possible for the ball. Legally, he cannot touch the ball until it reaches the top of the toss. Nor can he jump before the official releases the ball. But when he does jump he will rise faster than the ball. The player must practice to time his jump to reach the ball precisely as it reaches its peak height. This is not easy, especially since all officials throw the ball up slightly differently every time. But if the player has his technique down pat, he will have a chance to adapt to each jump-ball.

Most important is a pre-arrangement with your team-mates as to which direction the jumper is most likely to attempt to tap the ball. It does the jumper no good to get to the ball early if he merely taps it into a foe's hand.

Position is the single most important factor in successful rebounding. Whenever possible the player should take an inside position on his foe, with his back to him, facing the basket. Quickness can get you there first. You should block out the other player and be in a position to go for the ball yourself. You seek the position from which you are most apt to reach the ball. If you are a guard working outside, you look for the ball that will bounce hard outside off the hoop. If you are a forward, or a center, you look for the ball that must be taken right off the hoop, the moment it comes off the hoop, since you are not permitted to touch it while it is on the rim.

Always assume the shot will miss and there will be a rebound. Most shots will miss. If you're a guard and are inside, go for the ball. If you're outside, wait for the long rebound or the loose ball off a scramble, but be more concerned with getting back into defensive position if the other side rebounds the ball. If you're a for-

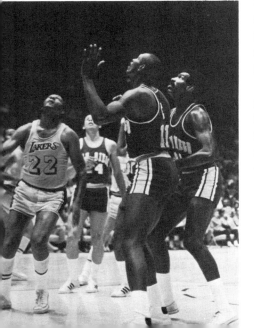

Here, everyone is standing around looking up. Is it a bird? Is it a plane? Is it Superstar? No, it's just a basketball and rebounders like Elgin Baylor (22), Elvin Hayes (11), and John Trapp are checking it out. (Photography, Inc.)

ward or center, go for the ball. Crouch, coil, and uncoil, springing up for the ball. It takes practice to time your jumps to reach the ball just as it comes off the hoop. It takes experience to anticipate the direction and trajectory different shots are apt to come off. But the more you observe shots closely, the better you will be able to judge them.

As with all defensive play, a lot of rebounding is sheer hard work and hustle and concentration. Because some players are stronger they can take and hold position better. Because some players are taller, can leap higher, or have better timing, they can reach the ball better. But the player can do a lot to take advantage of his strengths and play down his weaknesses. He can learn the moves his foes make to try to block him out. He can learn the type of shots his teammates and his foes take. The flatter the shot the harder and farther the rebound is apt to come. The shorter player can get inside on the taller player and make him reach over him. The player who looks for the rebound every time, who goes after it, is willing to fight for it, is going to get as many as he is physically capable of getting, which is all anyone can ask.

On defensive rebounds, grab the ball with both hands if at all possible. If you must reach for it with one hand, get the other hand on the ball as soon as possible. Tuck it into your gut with your elbows angled out. Come down with your feet spread wide. You can't use them as weapons, but jutting elbows and widespread legs discourage many defenders. When you come down, pivot away from your foe. Sometimes a quick dribble will free you from the defender. Be on the alert for an open teammate to pass to.

As you advance in ability in this area you may be able to come down with the ball while looking for a breaking teammate and be able to make the fast lead pass, possibly a football pass, that gets a fast-break going. The cen-

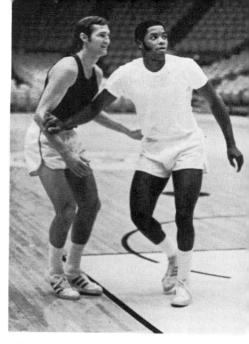

Taking position on me in practice, Jim McMillian is ready for a rebound. (Photography, Inc.)

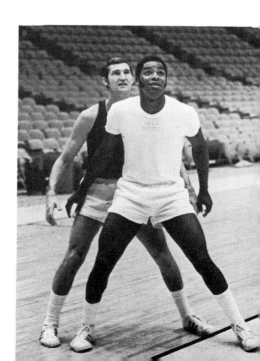

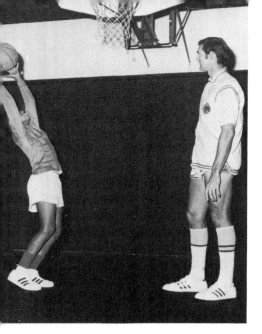

Kevin Hawkins comes down with a rebound in a garage session. Papa Tom was a great leaper and a fine rebounder. (Photography, Inc.)

ters who can do this are a tremendous help to a running team. Some cannot safely operate as swiftly as this maneuver demands. Jabbar, Wilt, and Unseld can get rid of the ball remarkably fast.

Our running game worked in the 1971-72 season because Wilt was the most effective rebounder in the league and really worked at making that fast outlet pass to get the fast-break going. We were not a big team but Wilt and Happy Hairston became the first two players on the same team in the same season to total more than 1,000 rebounds and they really did a job for us, especially in getting the ball and then getting rid of it to the fast-breakers.

However, the rebounder's first concern still must be simply getting the ball. I suspect that nearly as many baskets are scored on second and third shots as on first shots in each offensive thrust. Try not to let the other team shoot. Once they have shot, try to prevent their getting a follow-up shot.

The priorities are different in offensive rebounding. Here you are thinking offense more than defense. As you go up for the ball you must decide whether it would be best to tip it, to come down with it and then go back up for a short shot, or to come down and pass it off. If you make a mistake, the other team must still take the ball to the other end before it can score. However, possession of the ball is valuable at all times, so you shouldn't be careless with the possibilities. Often it is best to simply grab and protect the ball and begin a brand-new play. Hurried, off-balance offensive thrusts usually fail.

Whether on offense or defense, keep jumping for the ball until somone has secured the rebound. Very often the ball will still be bouncing around up there after the initial jump. Give it that second and third effort. If a defensive player grabs the rebound, don't hack at him in frustration and foul him, which happens far too often.

If he does not protect it properly, reach for it and try

to tie it up, forcing a jump-ball, or knock it or take it from him, but not in such a flailing fashion that you foul him. Right after coming down with a rebound, many players hold the ball in front of them, where it is vulnerable, so look for this. But if they protect it and you can't reach for it, revert to your defensive position. Try to discourage the fast pass that will launch the fast-break.

Rebounding is rough on the upper levels with giants crashing around in close quarters. The player must accept punishment as part of the job. On the lowest levels, most players just stand around waiting for the ball to come to them. Well, it's not very often going to come to you. You are going to have to go after it. And the aggressive player on the lower level who masters the techniques and goes after the ball is going to be a very valuable player.

Chamberlain, who is not far from 1,000 games played in the NBA and has never fouled out of a single game, holds two of the NBA rebound records, with 55 in one game (against Bill Russell's Boston team, no less) and 2,149 in one season, and overhauled the retired Russell's career record of 21,721 by reading 22,298 in 1972. Forwards Bob Pettit, Elgin Baylor, and Dolph Schayes rank next. Through the 1971-72 season, Wilt had won NBA rebounding honors eleven times. Russell won the rebounding crown four times. Still, big Bill always seemed to get the rebound when his team needed it.

Usually, if you are playing as aggressively as you should you will foul out of some games. Possibly Wilt could have been a bit more aggressive in his position, but he had such size and strength and such command of his position that he hasn't had to foul much. I must admit that I don't think they call the big glamour-guy centers for fouls as much as they do the guards. Those guys inside beat on each other and get away with murder while we're hustling around out in the open getting called for everything. It's just something we have to live with.

Jabbar has not totally mastered the art of rebound-

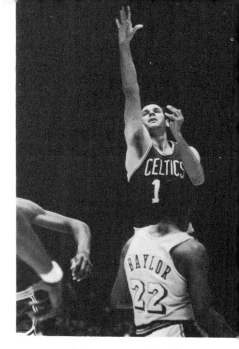

Two of the great offensive rebounders of a time are shown in action here. Above, Bailey Howell shoves a shot back up over Elgin Baylor; below, Elg shoves one up fro behind Bill Bradley (24) and Walt Frazier Dick Barnett watches. (Photography, Inc.)

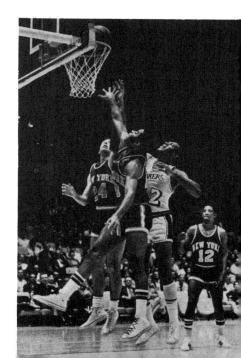

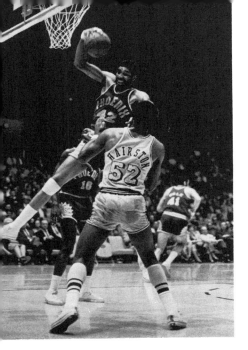

Grabbing a rebound by clasping his huge hand over the ball, Connie Hawkins awes Happy Hairston. Try it sometime. (Photography, Inc.)

Happiness is a guy named George, last name Wilson, as he smilingly sails down with a rebound. (Photography, Inc.)

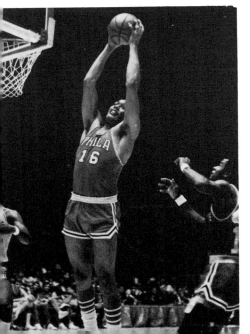

ing, but he has great timing and height and, as he gains weight and strength and becomes more aggressive, he may become awesome. At the moment, Wes Unseld, who at 6-7 or 6-8 is considerably shorter, is a bit tougher and a more effective rebounder. Elvin Hayes at 6-9 and Dave Cowens at 6-9 are almost as good. At times, 6-11 Nate Thurmond has been good, too, but he has often been handicapped by injuries. So has Willis Reed, another fine one. Mel Daniels and Artis Gilmore are outstanding.

Among forwards, Jerry Lucas, Bill Bridges, Happy Hairston, Connie Hawkins, Spencer Haywood, Gus Johnson, Billy Cunningham, Dave DeBusschere, Julius Erving, and Dan Issel are outstanding. Bailey Howell was probably the best offensive rebounder in the NBA. He could really put that ball back up there. Haywood has an advantage over others in that he actually has an extra joint on each finger. Really, where fingers have three divisions, his have four. He clamps on that ball with those claws. He and Hawkins smother the ball as though it were a grapefruit. Hawkins can catch the ball on top with one hand. Bridges and Johnson use muscle. Lucas, Cunningham, and DeBusschere use style. They all do the job.

Among guards, lanky Jerry Sloan, alert Walt Frazier, and springy Calvin Murphy are remarkable rebounders considering their position.

If you are going to play defense and get rebounds you are going to have to mix it up, learn techniques, master them, and work at using them. Work will pay off on defense more than in any other area of basketball. Without fine timing few players will become outstanding shooters. Fast reflexes help defenders, but desire and sweat will make up for a lot of flaws. And far more than most realize, many games are won on defense.

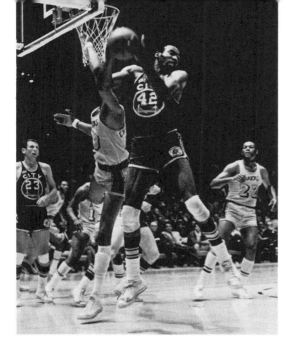

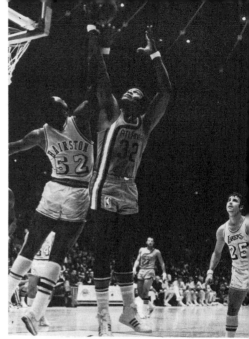

Four of the great rebounders are shown here in action. Above left is Nate Thurmond whipping Wilt, and right, Bill Bridges beating Happy Hairston. Below left is Wilt topping John Havlicek, and right, Elvin Hayes, without opposition. (Photography, Inc.)

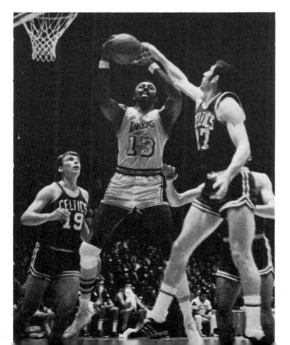

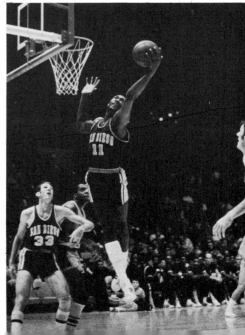

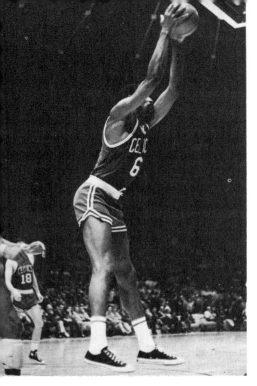

Big Bill Russell bags one of many he hauled
in while leading Boston to eleven world
titles in thirteen seasons. (Photography,
Inc.)

Bill Walton, UCLA's sophomore center
takes the ball off the board to display his
jumping ability.

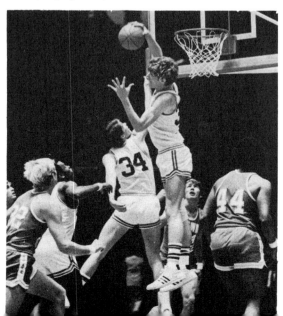

7. Strategy

Running flat-out, every muscle in my body at work, I tear around a block set up by Wilt Chamberlain, closely pursued by Joe Caldwell, Zelmo Beaty watching Wilt and ready to pick me up if necessary. We're working the pivot offense and I'm working to get free for a pass. It would do me no good to get in the right place for a shot if a defender is with me. The player actually handles the ball a small part of the time in any game. To a great extent, how he plays without the ball determines how good he is. Even though I don't have the ball here, Caldwell has to maintain defense on me. (Photography, Inc.)

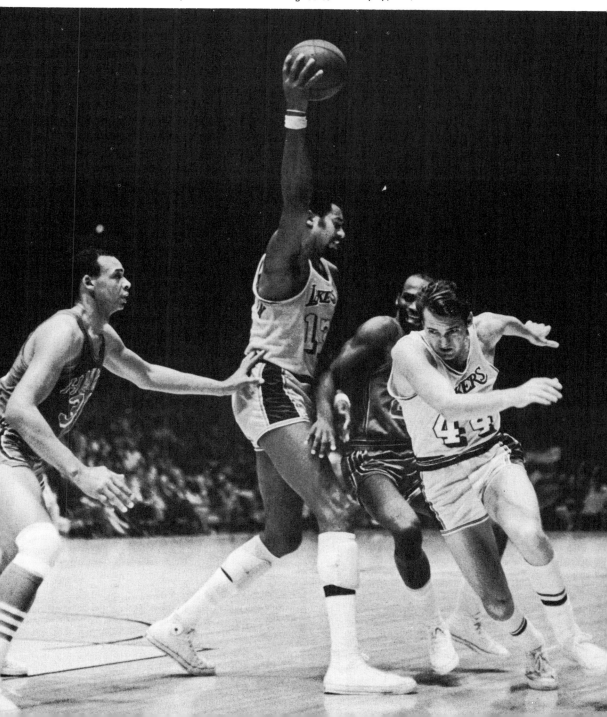

BASKETBALL is not a complicated game. Once the players learn the fundamentals and fit into a team, there is a lot of improvised activity. For example, a fast-break may erupt spontaneously. However, all improvisation is built on a firm base. It is based on dribbling, passing, and shooting techniques that have been practiced individually and rehearsed collectively. If the players don't know where to go, if they don't work with the other players, the break will fail. Also, it must grow out of a decision to run on offense. A team bent on pursuing a slow, pattern offense will often pass up the fast-break.

I am not a believer in inflexible systems and a lot of set plays. I believe a team should find a style of play that suits it but should practice various styles so it can try something else when the original plan isn't working. Players should have the freedom to operate within their style of play, but I believe it is handy to have a few set plays to use when its system is breaking down or to take advantage of certain openings.

I favor a running game and a man-to-man defense. But there are many variations of defense within the man-to-man style that must be mastered to give a team the variety it needs. And there are times when a zone is a very good defense to turn to on levels where it is permissible. I think you have to know how a zone operates on defense to combat it on offense. Essentially, I am saying that to use a clean, simple system on either offense or defense effectively the player and the team must have a knowledge of the various devices available. Strategy is making the best use of the tools available to you against a given team in a given situation.

First, you have to select your best lineup. This is the coach's job. If you have a pickup team without a coach, you should elect a player as captain who will make the decisions. Someone has to have the final say or all will be chaos. And don't elect a player on the basis of popularity. Vote for the boy you feel understands the game

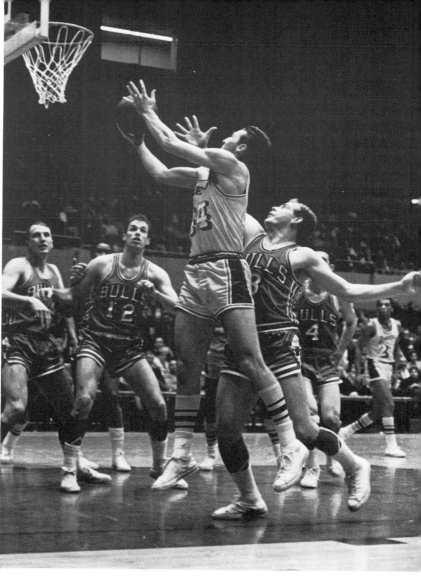

The defense is collapsing around me, but I have been sprung free in time to start a successful layup. (Photography, Inc.)

best, is most serious about it, and most fair. As much as possible, you want your five best men on the court. If the five are all small, you may wish to select a taller man to replace one of them. But only if he can do a job better than the otherwise more skilled player he replaces.

The decisions that must be made in this area are not easy ones. For example, I think everyone should try to win on all levels at all times, but there are practical rea-

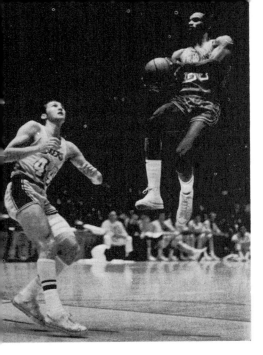

How high is up? How tall is tall? Joe Caldwell is 6-5 and can outjump some 7-footers. Here he must be 3 feet off the court as he goes up for a two-hand layup on me. I've arrived too late to go up with him. A fellow like Caldwell could play forward or even center on some teams better than some taller men playing the position. He is versatile and goes at forward or guard equally well. (Photography, Inc.)

sons why winning is not the only objective on the lower levels. I'd like to have a dime for every super player I've seen on lower levels who did not improve and every ordinary player who developed into a star later. The younger and less mature the boy is, the less clear his future. Thus you should never give up on a boy who is having his troubles but wants to improve. All boys can improve. Not all will become stars, however. It is very important on the lower levels to use as many boys as much as possible. And sometimes you have to take chances with a boy at an early stage who can be brought along to help you later.

Often, the tall player who may have shot up so fast he is more frail and awkward than other players is used because his height will give him a built-in advantage and he will not have to develop his talents as fully. However, one of my pet complaints is that too much emphasis is placed on the big man. I am not saying too much emphasis is placed on the outstanding big man. They dominate games as no little man ever could. But I think too many tall players get the edge when roster cuts are being made and starting lineups selected. Often, there are smaller players who can do the same job better. Skill can make up for a number of inches in height. I think the pros are the most guilty in this respect. I consider quickness and ability to be the most important talents a player can have, far more important than height. Sometimes a small boy gets beaten by a bigger man on offense and the coach will say, "Well, he's just not big enough," but will forget the steals the smaller man made on the bigger man.

Basically, you begin by looking for your center. If a shorter man is a better leaper and a better rebounder, he may well be preferable. Ballhandling is very important for a center, as a lot of plays are run off the pivot. And strength is important because he has to be able to get position on his opposing pivot in close to the basket.

The biggest problem the center has over players in other positions is that he must play most of the game with his back to the basket. The center has to be aware of this and concentrate on getting a feel for the court and its markings so he knows where he is in relation to the basket. Often, he is going to have to pivot around and make a quick move toward the basket.

The pivot must master a lot of in-close shots. He doesn't have to shoot outside set-shots or even very many jumpers, but he should have a good hook shot. He should work especially hard on setting up picks, as he is going to serve as a blocker for other players' shots and drives. He should be able to make the "football" pass and the "handoff" skillfully.

Agility is so important in the pivot position that on many lower levels a short player who is by far the best player on court goes into the center slot and completely outclasses his foe. I think it is much harder for a bigger man to cover a smaller man in any position than it is for a smaller man to cover a bigger man. This is because the smaller men are usually quicker and more agile. You can't underestimate the advantage of height in this game, but you can't underestimate the advantage of quickness and agility, either.

Bill Russell represented the ideal center. He was only a fair shooter, but he could get baskets when he needed them. He was a great rebounder, defender, and shot-blocker, a superb passer, and he orchestrated games beautifully. "Orchestrate" is the word he uses. And by it he means he set the tempo and saw that all his team-mates got to do as much as possible the things they did best. He made all his teammates better by helping them to realize their potential. His record speaks for itself. He not only was the most valuable player I've ever known in basketball, but probably the most valuable in any sport in my time.

Which is not to put down Wilt Chamberlain, who has

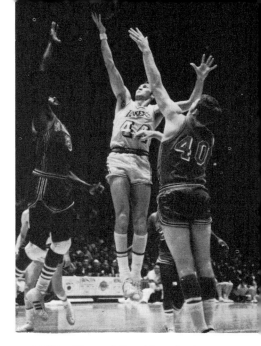

At 6-3, with a well-timed leap, I get up over a much taller player such as 6-11 Walt Bellamy, left. Jumping ability and long arms add inches to my actual height. (Photography, Inc.)

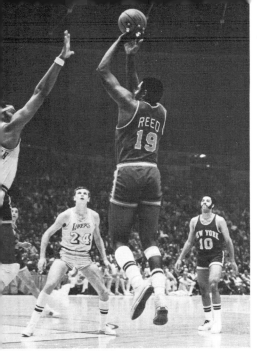

A picture-perfect all-around center, Willis Reed goes up to pop in a one-hander over Wilt Chamberlain with Keith Erickson and Walt Frazier watching. Reed is not brilliant in any one area, although he has classic shooting style, but he does everything a center should do, and does it all well. (Photography, Inc.)

been a far superior scorer, the greatest point-maker the game has ever known, possibly a better rebounder. Russell's teams won more championships, but I'm not sure they won more games. Wilt's teams won a lot of games and a lot of divisional titles. To put him down because his teams did not win more league championship play-offs would be to put myself down because my teams won less. No player was ever more dominant than Wilt in 1972. He became a classic center. He did whatever had to be done to win.

I think centers are more responsible than guards in the winning of crowns because they are more dominant in games, but a lot enters into the winning of championships and it is difficult to hang it on one man. Many feel Jabbar will become the sort of winner Russell was. He was in college and won the pro crown in his second season, but he could not carry his club to the title in the 1971-72 season when his key aide, Oscar Robertson, was injured, and he has a long, long way to go to match Russell's pro statistics. Like Bill he is a tremendously smart and unselfish player, who gets the most from his teams. And he is the quickest and most agile big man I've seen.

Willis Reed has been an outstanding center who has been handicapped by injuries. But he has classic shooting style, good all-around ability, and an unselfish sense of team play. Nate Thurmond is another who has been handicapped by injuries, but he may be the most underrated player of recent years. He sacrifices for his team. He is a tremendous defender and rebounder and a skilled and versatile performer. Dave Cowens came a long way in the 1971-72 season. Special mention should be made of Wes Unseld, who at around 6-7 is the smallest center in the league, but still one of the best. He is unselfish, smart, and powerful. He rebounds well and gets the ball out amazingly fast. The ABA developed a center in this class in the great Artis Gilmore.

The forwards must have good size and good strength. They must operate in congested corners and must move into the tight middle. They need fair shooting variety and range. It is, frankly, an easier position to play than guard. The forward doesn't have to bring the ball up-court. He is passed to more than passing. And he has shorter shots to make than guards. Still, the cornerman who can play his position right can be just as important to his team as any guard. He is in close to the hoop and is asked to do a lot of scoring and rebounding. Also, he can make up for the center's deficiencies.

Years ago in pro ball, 6-5 was about the right height for a cornerman. Elgin Baylor was 6-5. Now you have guards who are 6-5 and cornermen who are 6-8 and 6-10, and sometimes they're 7-footers. Size and agility are more important than speed here. Bob Pettit and Dolph Schayes were not fast, but they were strong and deter-mined and were two of the best cornermen ever to play this game. All-around, Elgin Baylor was the best. Rick Barry is about the best scoring forward I've faced. Billy Cunningham, Connie Hawkins, Julius Erving, Spencer Haywood, and Bob Love are fine offensive cornermen. Jerry Lucas, Gus Johnson, and Dave DeBusschere are brilliant all-around cornermen. Lucas played center ef-fectively in the 1971-72 season, but he's a forward.

All-time I'll put Baylor and Barry up front with Rus-sell in the center. Wilt could be there, too, of course. In the backcourt I'll put Oscar Robertson. It's tough to pick one man with him. Maybe Dave Bing. Walt Frazier is right there, too. Robertson is a great all-around back-courtman. K. C. Jones was the best defensive-styled guard. Bob Cousy was the best all-around ballhandler. Gail Goodrich, Dave Bing and Walt Frazier are the best young guards in basketball today, and getting better every year. One-on-one, Earl Monroe is, I think, the sin-gle most exciting player in basketball today. John Havlicek, who also plays forward, is exceptional.

Although size helps anywhere, it's quickness and ball-handling ability you look for in guards. Every team needs at least one player to bring the ball upcourt and

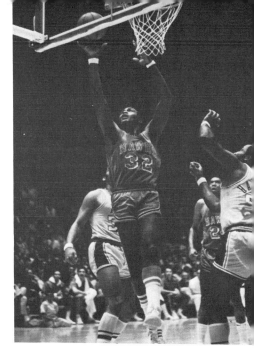

A good-sized rugged cornerman, Bill Brid-ges, goes up to haul in a rebound. Bill is a tough rebounder and defender, an under-rated all-around performer. (Photography, Inc.)

Quick and agile, Billy Cunningham, one of the fine forwards, goes high against Keith Erickson. (Photography, Inc.)

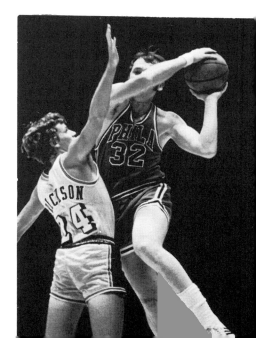

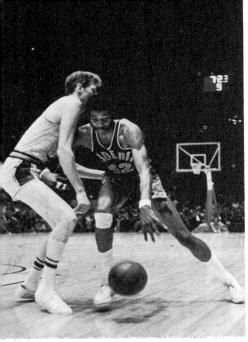

Versatile Connie Hawkins at 6-8 works on 7-foot Mel Counts. A center in his youth, a center part of his early pro days, he now has settled down at forward, but he could play almost any position because of his agility, ballhandling, and jumping ability. (Photography, Inc.)

get the play going. And it doesn't matter if he isn't a great shooter. I've seen teams on the lower levels severely handicapped because they were playing their five biggest men or best shooters and had no one to handle the ball.

Look for the big fellow who gets up the highest and handles himself best in the pivot. Look for two good-sized but agile cornermen. If one is very good offensively and the other very good defensively, perfect. Look for two quick, clever backcourtmen. If one is a good ball-handler and the other a good outside shooter, perfect.

If you have a good player left over, let him come off the bench. Use him. The sixth man as pioneered by Red Auerbach in Boston with first Frank Ramsey, then John Havlicek, can be enormously valuable. There were times they were better than the starters, but they were more valuable coming off the bench, stirring things up, giving the team new pep, picking up a couple of quick baskets. Dick Barnett did this job brilliantly for the Lakers until traded. Cazzie Russell did it brilliantly for the Knicks until traded. Clearly, such players are underrated.

Size simply should not be the determining factor in making position decisions. As good a center as could be, Russell was not the biggest. Nor was the best forward, Baylor. Sometimes a taller man is better suited for a corner, a smaller man for the pivot. Often a much smaller backcourtman can do a better job than the man picked over him.

Basketball intelligence is tremendously important in a backcourtman. To a great extent he controls the flow of a game. With experience, I have learned to speed things up or slow things down, get the team to doing one thing or another, and it has increased my value enormously. Defensive ability is tremendously important in all positions. Look for the players who can hamper the opposition as well as those who can shoot. You should have at least one up front and one in the backcourt to cover the other club's top offensive threats.

Court balance is critical. Obviously, every player is not as good as every other player. If you have a weak position, try to pair it with a strong position. If your fifth player is a guard and very weak, try to have one of your better players complement him at guard.

I think players should learn as many positions as possible. The younger they are the less they can know how they will grow and how their talents will develop. And it always helps to be flexible. Many of today's star guards and forwards were centers in high school when they may have been the biggest men on their teams. I was a for-

Possibly the most versatile of players in recent years, John Havlicek flips one up backhanded as West, Don Nelson, and Happy Hairston watch. For years Havlicek was not a starter for Boston simply because he was so explosive coming off the bench. He plays guard or forward equally well and is one of the truly tireless performers in basketball today. In playoffs he has gone whole games without showing the slightest sign of weariness. He is perfectly conditioned, always ready, and as good a competitor as I've faced. (Photography, Inc.)

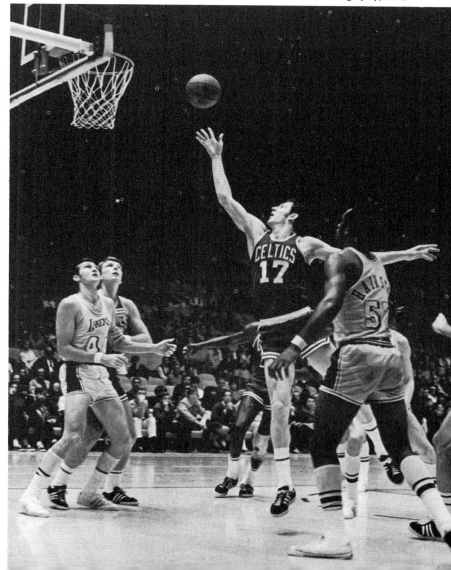

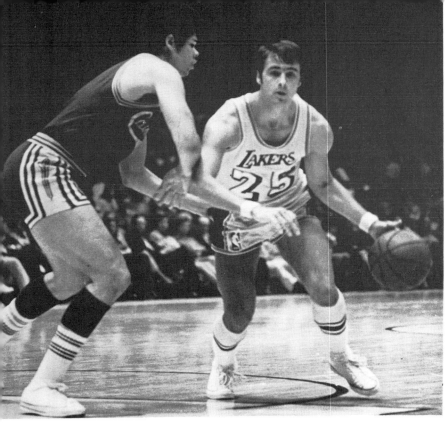

A strong runner, an explosive performer in John Wooden's fast-break offense and pressing defense at UCLA, Gail Goodrich is the sort of little man who helps make a running game go. At 6-1, Gail gives away inches to almost all his rivals, but natural talents and determination have made him a top pro. (Photography, Inc.)

ward until I got into pro ball and was converted to the backcourt. A fellow like John Havlicek, who can play forward and guard equally well, is tremendously valuable to his team. Pat Riley does this for us. Jerry Lucas went to center from forward on the Knicks and did a job for them. Learn as many positions as possible and eventually you'll fit into your best one.

Sometimes players must sacrifice for the good of their teams. A fellow whose future may be at guard may have to play forward or even center because his team needs him there most, possibly because he may be bigger than others on the club. Accept it. It will help you in the long run. And how good you are is not nearly as important as how much you help your team.

On offense, practice both a running, fast-breaking game and a slowdown, pattern style. A good team must be able to go to either. One of the most effective parts of the Milwaukee Bucks success story is that they can shift fluidly from one type of game to another and play both equally well.

Basically, the smaller your team the more you should run. The faster your players, the more you should run. A big team that can control the ball a lot can use a control style of offense effectively. If you have a big man who can hardly run, it will be difficult to fast-break, even if you have four fast men. The smaller the team the more aggressive it's going to have to play. It's going to have to steal the ball a lot and penetrate with swift passing and drives on offense to combat taller clubs.

In the fast-break, of course, every player is moving and the ball is worked upcourt as rapidly as possible and passed up to the middleman and on to the lead man as often as possible. All of the players must keep running, but not, I might add, to the basket. Only the lead man should go to the basket. But once he shoots, others should follow him for possible follow-up shots. The offense must be spread to permit fluid movement. Thus the forwards go into the corners. If a guard is upcourt on the fast-break, a forward fills his position in the backcourt. Balance and spread are maintained. One trailer must hang back to protect defensively against a turnover.

An aggressive attack tends to upset most foes. However, if the other team has faster, surer, or generally better personnel than you do, you'd better slow things down and use a careful style of offense. Never overrate your foes, but never underestimate them, either. Take a realistic view of the club you are opposing, what they can and cannot do best. As much as possible, be aware of what you have to do to handle the other club best. As much as possible, try to get them to play your game. If you are a small, swift, club, try to get them into a running game. But if it's not working, don't be afraid to try something else.

Admitting to yourself that the other club has better personnel is not the same as giving up. Almost any team can win any given game. And the team that plays the smartest game will win about as often as the superior team. Actually, the smartest team is the superior team. If the other team is bigger and stronger, play a controlled offense. Slow the pace, but work the ball as fast as you can, looking for the good shots, trying to spring open the best shooters. The team that loses a lot of rebounds will get few second shots and must make every shot count.

If you have a tall man, one solid, controlled offense is to play off the pivot. The ball is fed into the center and the other players weave and cut off him, looking to get the ball in the open or off a screen. Once you have set

Working the pivot offense, Bill Russell prepares to hand off a short pass to John Havlicek, cutting off him. Wilt is watching Bill, but Tom Hawkins and Keith Erickson have been trapped behind Sam Jones, so if Wilt picks up Havlicek, Russell will be freed for a return pass and open shot. (Photography, Inc.)

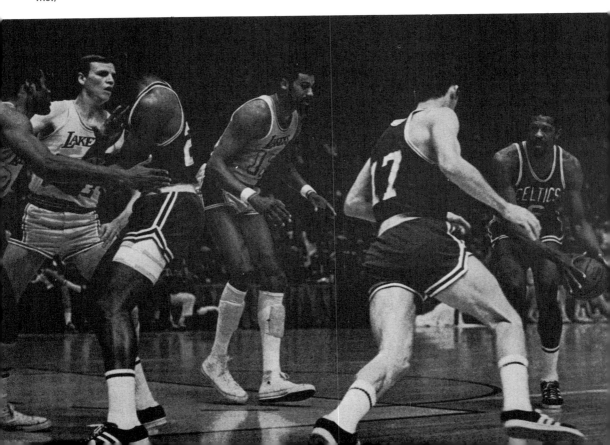

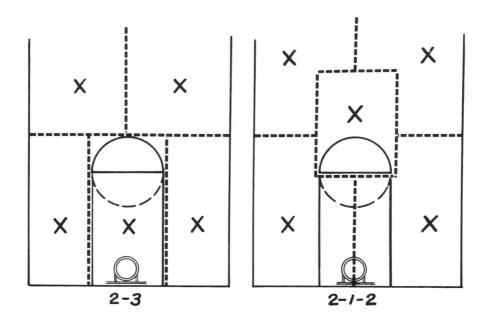

2-3

2-1-2

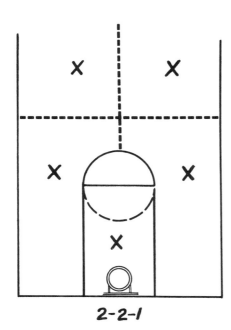

2-2-1

OFFENSIVE ZONES

up and are working the ball in the offensive zone, all teams, even those that are fast-breaking teams, are in a controlled offense. It is critical that the players without the ball keep moving in a pattern. They must be looking for openings without, to put it bluntly, crashing into one another. This takes practice. With two tall men, a double-pivot may be set up to spread the offense farther.

Every player must know where he is going to go and where his teammates are going to go. The players who handle the ball best should handle it most. The players who shoot it best should shoot it most. The players must know the positions from which their teammates shoot best. When they spot them in those spots they should try to give them the ball. If the other team has a weak player or a player in foul trouble, work on this position, send players through this position with the ball.

Once you are setting up in the offensive zone, there are a number of offensive patterns you may take, some of which are drawn in this chapter. Pick the pattern that best suits your personnel and lean to it, but don't be afraid to shift into another pattern periodically to unsettle the opposition. Use numbers or colors to denote each pattern and let your "quarterback," usually a designated guard, call them out when a change is called for.

Very often the first shot that presents itself is not the best shot. Look for the percentage shots. When your good shot comes up, take it. A lot of young players are hesitant, overly modest. If it's a shot you can hit four or five times out of ten, take it. Don't force your shot. Take all the time you need. There'll be no time-limit imposed on you until you get into AAU, Olympic, or pro ball, and by then you'll be psychologically ready to handle it. In the meantime, don't be afraid to move the ball back out and start all over again.

I prefer the running, fast-breaking game, especially on the lower levels. If it is run well it puts tremendous pressure on the other clubs. Once you are set up I favor a

OFFENSE "YELLOW"

1 and 5 move out to clear the side. 3 clears defense and cuts out of the middle. 4 moves up to fake screen for 2, then rolls out and takes bounce pass.

OFFENSE "BLUE"

1 passes to 3, then circles left. 5 and 4 circle to left, cleaning out right side. 2 cuts off 3, takes short pass, and shoots off his screen.

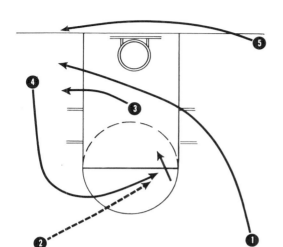

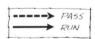

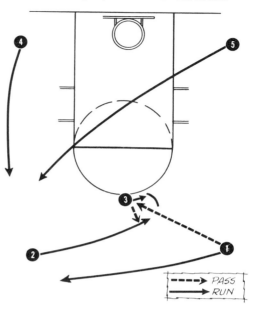

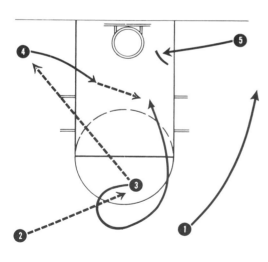

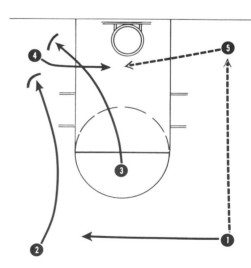

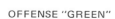

OFFENSE "GREEN"

1 moves out of play to right. 2 passes to 3, who passes to 4 and circles. 4 drives toward basket, but quickly passes to 3, who has circled back, moved behind screen set by 5, and is open for short shot.

OFFENSE "RED"

2 and 3 set up screens on left side. 1 passes to 5 and clears out. 4 cuts between screen and takes pass at basket from 5.

pivot offense. I like to see the ball in with the center if he is a good ballhandler, because once the ball is in close to the basket you are a great threat to score and have placed a lot of pressure on the defense.

When you are not able to fast-break or are stalled because the other club has set up swiftly on defense, I believe in a free-lance game off that pivot offense. For years, frankly, the Laker game was to give the ball to Elg or myself and let us work all alone for a shot. It worked to some extent, but in the end it didn't work. We could only do so much alone. We were taking the other guys out of the game. You should use as many men as possible in your offensive flow.

There are basic plays a team uses in a free-lance offense up front, such as the pivot play in which you work off the center, and the give-and-go in which a breaking player gives the ball to a teammate and goes for the basket, looking for a return pass. I don't believe in using too many set plays. I think imposing a lot of X's and O's on a player takes away his individuality. If he has to go to certain places in certain ways every time, he may not be able to do those things he does best.

However, a smart coach can shape plays to take advantage of the things his players do best. All teams need set plays for certain situations. Again, these can be coded by color or number, and the quarterback can call them out as needed—on instructions from the coach. Some of these plays are illustrated in this book. One of the strengths of my Lakers in 1971-72 was we could work a lot of different offenses.

Figure out your foe's defense as soon as possible. This is not as easy as it sounds. Many defenses are concealed and may not show up for a few plays. You can usually determine if a team is in a zone defense by sending a man through the middle. If no one follows him all the way through, the other team is using a zone.

If the other team is congesting the area under the

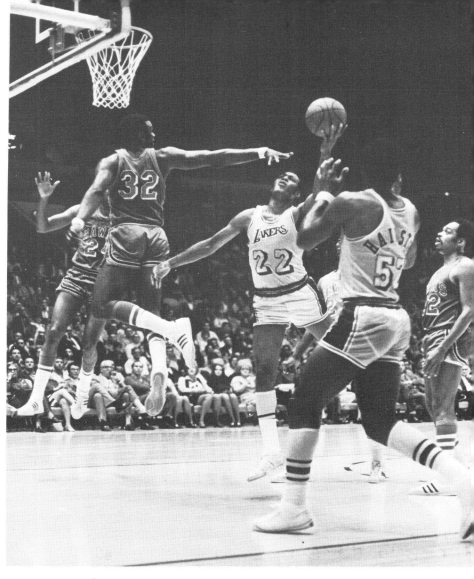

backboard, open it up if possible. Pull your pivot from a low post (almost directly under the basket) to a high post (out near the free-throw line). If your center can shoot from outside it is helpful to let him do so for a while to lure a good rebounding center out from under the basket.

The fast-break is a good offense against a team that plays a good man-to-man defense. It gets fast movement

Caught in the switches, Bill Bridges sticks out a hand to trouble Elgin Baylor, but Bill's teammates have lost the play on defense and Happy Hairston is open for a pass and an easy layup if Elg feeds off to him. (Photography, Inc.)

going against the defenders and makes more of an offensive threat of the lesser shooters on your club, since it may free them for easy shots. In working on a good man-to-man offense, use a lot of screens and force your foes into as many switches as possible. Work on the weakest link in a man-to-man defense. Try to force mismatches on switches. Drive a big forward off an outside screen toward a smaller man who must pick him up and can be carried toward the basket with him. Work "figure-eight" weaves, which are described in the following chapter, on practice.

You can fast-break against a good zone defense, especially before the defense has set up. Once the defense has set up, even if a defensive player loses his man he is going to be picked up as he enters the next zone. Do not dribble much against a zone. Try to penetrate it with fast passing. Return passes to the passer often and fast, as the zone moves with the ball, freeing briefly the man who has just given up the ball. Shoot over the zone to try to bring it out and loosen it up. Work on the zone of

A fast-break is underway, Wilt Chamberlain having rebounded and fed off to Elgin Baylor, who is dribbling upcourt as Boston defenders Bailey Howell, Em Bryant, and Bill Russell turn to race back and cover up. (Photography, Inc.)

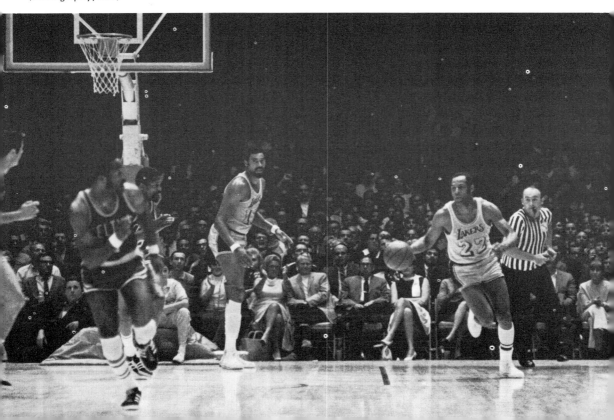

a weak defender. Overload a specific zone by pouring a second or third man into it.

One big advantage to a good fast-break is that it tends to disrupt the other team's offense as well as its defense. The other side will be reluctant to penetrate with many players for fear of being caught without potential defenders to pick up a fast-break that may develop.

With the fast-break a team can pick up points in bunches—6, 8, 10 points in a hurry—to make up deficits and demoralize the other club. There is nothing more discouraging to a team than to work hard a long time for one good, careful shot, then to have the other team get it back, bang-bang.

The main disadvantage to the fast-break is that it is run fast and so leads to mistakes. Offensive turnovers hurt any team's chances, and to work hard to get the ball and then throw it away is demoralizing. The faster you move the more you're apt to make mistakes. Just running is no advantage if it does not lead to baskets. All teams are going to make mistakes. They must not get discouraged by them. But if they make too many they must try to discover what they are doing wrong. They may be moving too fast for their own abilities.

Aggressiveness will make up for some mistakes. Lack of aggressiveness costs more teams more games than mistakes. But a balance must be sought. The team should play as aggressively as it can, but not to the point where it makes too many mistakes.

A good, aggressive man-to-man defense works with a fast-break offense. You will get a lot of steals and loose balls on defense that will lead to breaks. If you are running on offense it is good to be running on defense.

It is possible to combine a zone defense with a fast-break offense or a pressing defense with a control offense. In any event, you must choose your offense by the defense you want to use and vice versa.

There are many defenses teams can use, including

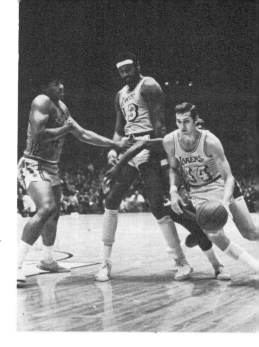

Cutting off a pick placed down by Wilt, I elude Monroe but Wes Unseld seems to be flexing a muscle as though to pick me up and maybe knock my block off. (Photography, Inc.)

An aggressive, pressing defense is applied on me here. Was a foul called? I hope so. (Photography, Inc.)

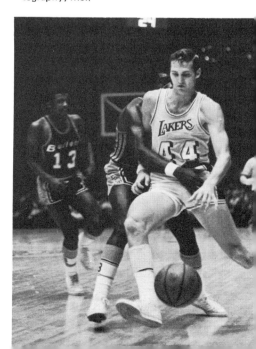

zones, which are illustrated on these pages. I am not a great believer in zone defenses, but there are sound basketball men who favor them and the young player must learn them, because he is usually going to use some prior to reaching the pro level.

In the zone, each player is responsible defensively for an area of the court. He follows the ball and adjusts his position within his area according to where the ball goes. When a man enters his zone the defender picks him up. When two or more enter his zone he picks up, first, the man with the ball, and second, the man nearest the goal. The zone defender tends to adopt a higher stance with his hands held higher and moving more than the man-to-man defender, whose posture is governed more by his man's moves. He is as responsible for the ball as he is for men. He must try to deflect balls that are thrown through his area.

There are many advantages to the zone. It's good to use until players have mastered man-to-man defense. With a zone you can get the smaller players farther away from the basket and they are not going to be drawn into mismatches under the hoop. It is also an effective defense for a team that has one outstanding big man. You want him under the basket at all times, to block shots or grab rebounds. Thus many teams presumably using man-to-man defenses are using one-man zones in that they have big centers who never leave the basket area.

However, in the long run a zone is easier to beat than a man-to-man run with equal efficiency. A good team can overload zones, pass through zones, shoot over them, take them apart systematically. I said a good team. A bad team will often be beaten badly by a zone. Of course, a bad team may be beaten badly by anything. But a good team is usually troubled more by one or more variations on a good man-to-man defense.

The man-to-man defense can be played many ways. It may be played loosely. In a sense, this is a careful de-

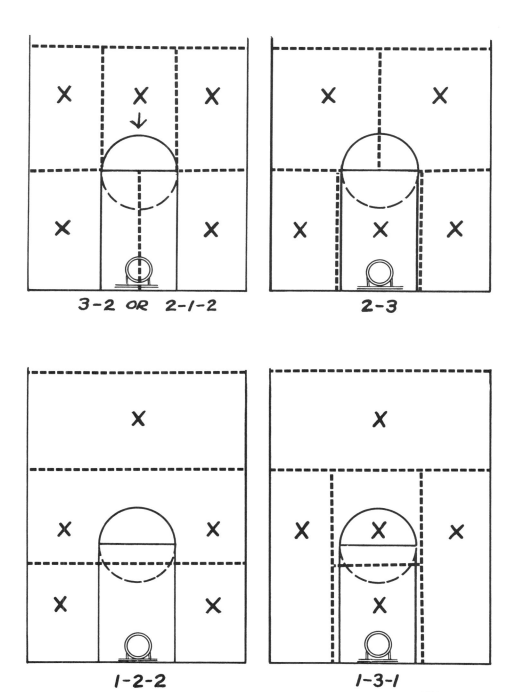

3-2 OR 2-1-2

2-3

1-2-2

1-3-1

ZONE DEFENSES

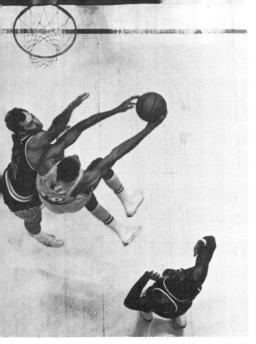

Playing a one-man zone, Jim Fox was hanging around the hoop, in position to pick up a forward, Bill Hewitt, who had lost his man and was driving for a layup in this photo taken from overhead. (Photography, Inc.)

Double-teamed by guard Gail Goodrich (25) and forward Happy Hairston, Hal Greer, one of the great guards and an underrated player, is trapped on his dribble. The veteran became one of the rare players past a career of 20,000 points during his thirteenth pro season, 1970-71. (Photography, Inc.)

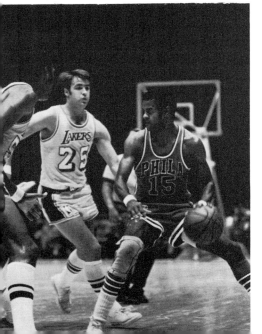

fense. The defense is not overplaying and is not going to make a lot of mistakes, and it is playing against the possible drive as much as against the possible shot. The man-to-man may be played tightly, in which case the defenders stay close to their men. This is a good way if you have quick defenders or the other team has poor ballhandlers. A step removed from this is a press, in which the defense is not merely tight on the attackers but all over them. Unless your whole defensive strategy is based on your having small, quick players, the pressing defense should be used only when you need the ball badly, because you are overplaying and gambling and risking a lot of fouls.

The press may be applied full-court or only from midcourt. A team may apply a zone-press, in which the press is applied only at the other end of the court, at midcourt, or near the basket. Basically, you are seeking to disrupt your foes' offensive rhythm. Soon they will be unsure which way you are coming at them or how. A half-court press is a good defensive tactic, as it enables the defense to size up the offense before going to work and saves considerable energy.

With man-to-man defenses you are going to have to use a switching system. There must be a cover-up for the mistake or failure of any player, and the switch is it. The man closest to the loose man has to pick him up. The defensive center even must leave the offensive center to pick up a guard's man. The secret to the success of any switching defense lies in the switcher picking up the man swiftly and someone else, usually the man who has lost his own, picking up the switcher's man.

Out of a man-to-man defense, double-teaming may be emphasized. A player guarding a weak man may tend to slide off him a lot to add to a teammate's defense of another player. A team may wish to put two men on an outstanding foe as much as possible and does so by having whoever is closer to him join the normal defender. If

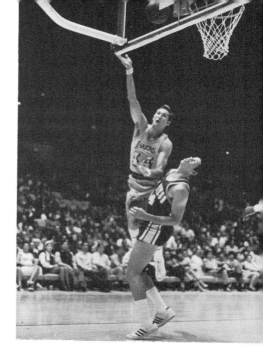

the star is the opposing center the defense may collapse around him. In this defense the defenders tend to draw inward, and whenever the ball looks like it is going to the pivot or is thrown to him, they drop off their men a bit and slide toward the center.

There are many combinations of defenses teams may use. One very effective for teams with one quick, outstanding defender and otherwise ordinary personnel is to use a four-man zone with the one defender as a free-lancer, pursuing the ball and the ballhandler at all times. This, in effect, pressures and double-teams the ballhandler. It is especially effective in the backcourt, where the play originates. The free-lancer tends to get a lot of steals and forces bad passes.

The team simply must assess its own personnel and decide which defense it is going to use depending on the offense it is going to face. Facing a team which uses a lot of blocks and screens, you must switch a lot. If you are losing your men a lot on a fast-break, if you need the ball badly, turn to a press. If you have five small, but fast men, use the press anyway.

Think things out. If a team is running a lot, but is not attacking effectively, let 'em run. Worry only about those things that are working for the other side. But permit the pattern to develop before altering your basic, favored style. Don't panic because the other side works something once or twice. Avoid making too many changes. Change to confuse your foes, not yourselves.

Build your defense to prevent giving away the easy basket to the other side. Make them work for every point they get. And lend emphasis to putting pressure on the other club's best player. On the lower levels, if you stop the other team's best player, you usually will win. The higher level you reach, the more good players the other team will have and the more dangerous it will be to concentrate on any one man.

If you have more than one good player and the other

Driving for a layup, I am blocked out and forced up and over a defender. The position of the defender's feet indicates he was moving when he got in my way, so the foul should have been called on him. In any situation, the man screening or blocking must take his position and hold it to be entitled to it. He cannot move into another man's path as the man gets there. (Photography, Inc.)

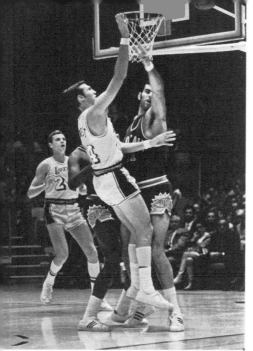

Picked up by two men as I reach the basket,
I get the ball batted away by big pivot Neal
Walk. (Photography, Inc.)

team is defensing your best player with extra pressure
and double-teams, take advantage of this. Any time the
other side has two men on one man, you have one man
without anyone on him. Work to get a good man in that
position. Send the good man through the vacated territory.

If you have a hot man, feed him. Take advantage of
his streak until it runs out or until the other team begins
to overload on him. When they do, decoy him and go to
someone else.

Logic dictates many of these moves, but many teams
do not play logically. They do not concentrate on what
is developing on court. They may be inflexible. Think
things out. Know the situation at all times. You don't
have to know the score, just the margin. Are you even?
Ahead or behind? By how much? How much time is
left? If you have the lead with time running out in a
period, play for the last shot.

Try to keep your cool. If something is working for
you, stay with it. Don't switch from a successful fast-
break to a slow-down game just because you've built a
lead. Wait until the fast-break isn't working for you any
longer. I've seen many teams fall apart when they
stopped running and tried to sit on a lead. Sometimes
when you stop doing a certain thing, it is difficult to get
back the rhythm to resume it. Stick with whatever is
successful. Play the game that is working for you. If you
have to overcome a deficit, try to apply increasing pressure without rushing. Keep chipping away. Don't try to
do it all at once. Don't turn to desperate things you
don't do very well.

First, do those things on offense and defense you do
best. Second, and only second, fit them to combat the
things the other team does best. Try to get the other
team to play your game rather than altering your own.
In selecting both an offense and defense, consider the
size and individual abilities of your personnel before you

worry about what the other team can and can't do. You
must coordinate the right offense to the right defense
and vice versa.

Keep things simple. It is better to practice to points
of perfection a few things than it is to have a lot of
things you do, but do badly. Work on building up your
varieties and abilities in practice and put them into
games as you reach a reasonable level of perfection with
them.

On both offense and defense, first select a system
that puts as many players as possible into the play as
effectively as possible. Then, and only then, build up the
roles of your best players.

Seek a system of offense that will not only free your
best players for their best shots, but your other players
for their best shots, too. As much as possible, make it a
five-man team that highlights your best players rather
than a one-man team that shadows your lesser players.

On defense, select a system that will work best for
the whole team, concealing the weaknesses of those who
are weak defensively.

On offense, stress court balance and penetration. The
easy shot by any player is almost always better than the
hard shot by your best shooter. I'd rather break anyone
in for a free layup than to take my best outside jump-
shot. I may hit half or more of those outside jumpers,
but most players can make nine out of ten open layups.
Look to get the ball in as close to the bucket as possible.
Don't overpass. Don't pass up good shots. Sometimes it
helps open up the basket area to the easy shot with outside shooting. But look to open up that basket area to
penetration.

On defense, stress court balance and rebounding. The
best defense is control of the ball. If you have the ball
the other side can't score. When you don't have it, try to
steal it. But not if you have to gamble to the point

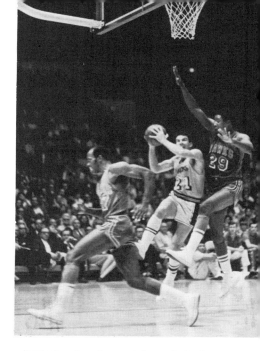

Exploding for a layup at the end of a fast-
break, Johnny Egan has foes Paul Silas and
Joe Caldwell flying past him in their rush to
cover up. (Photography, Inc.)

where you'll give them openings and easy shots. You will get the ball a lot more often by rebounding than by stealing.

The most important thing is to give your opponent the worst possible shot and, if possible, only one shot on each series. If you take the second shot away from most teams you'll win most games. If the other team has only one good player and you can stop him, you'll usually win. On the other hand, rarely can one man beat you alone. If the other team has a man you can't stop, work on stopping the rest of his team. Don't give him a thing, but don't destroy the balance of your defense to stop a single man.

Play smart. Your brain is as much a weapon as your legs and your arms. Think things out. Don't just watch games to see who wins. See what the men who play your position do, and what their defenders do, and what works and what doesn't work. Try to figure out why. Try to figure out the offensive and defensive patterns, and how they're applied, and why they succeed or fail. Try to decide what you would do in different situations. When you get involved in a game, try to learn why things are happening as they are and try to prolong the favorable things and curtail the unfavorable things.

Primarily, it is concentration and experience. Even the fan will find he gets increased pleasure from a game if he understands its inner workings, the many games played within a game. As a player you are expected to understand your sport so you can use sound strategy to complement whatever physical abilities you possess. Seldom are things as they appear on the surface. Behind the statistics of the superstar, there are strengths and weaknesses, things he does well and things he does not do well. Beneath the shell of every player there are secrets he strives to keep. Does he avoid going one way or another? Does he make careless passes? Does he tire fast? Is he discouraged by rough play? Are you? Try to understand your own strengths and weaknesses, your own tendencies.

Get to know yourself, your game, the game, the way others play it. Play smart.

8. Practice

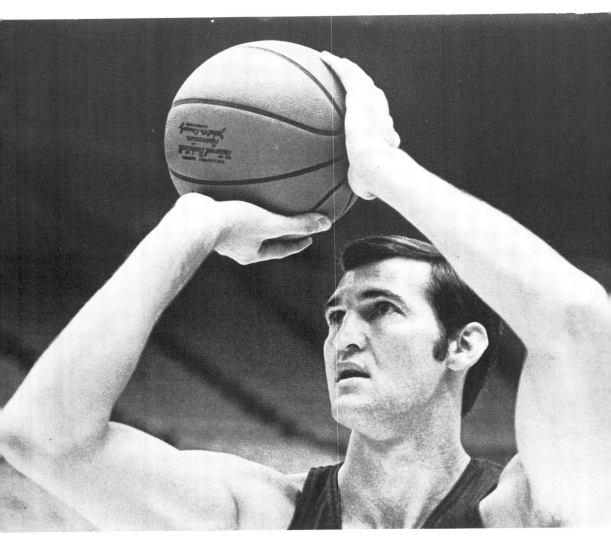

Practicing my one-hand shot, my posture is pictured here. The ball is held just above my head, on the pads of my hand, wrist cocked well back, elbow pointed at the basket, my free hand holding the ball steady until the release. (Photography, Inc.)

MOST OF your career, practice will be as important as playing. For the most part you'll play as well as you practice. In games you will only be able to use effectively those things you have practiced enough to do well. You'll put in a lot less time playing games than you will practicing your game. Don't put it down. Don't underestimate its importance. Look forward to it as you do games.

As you get older, practice will become harder to endure. As I passed into my thirties, after years of playing as a boy, after four years playing in high school, after four years playing in college, after ten years playing as a pro and more, I had less energy to spare. Yet, even now, I enjoy practice, in some ways as much as games. In practice you can be loose. There's no pressure on you. Not so in games.

And you never stop learning, you really never do. If you are very good, sheer talent will carry you a long way. However, as you step up in class, you'll have to learn new techniques. As long as I've played, there is always someone who can show me new tricks.

As you go along, there are new coaches and new teammates, new styles to learn and adjust to. As you get older you must find ways of doing things differently to make up for some quickness you have lost or to save you precious stamina. The thinking part of the game keeps growing. There's always someone who comes along to show me a new wrinkle.

Practice is precious. Treasure it. Make good use of it. The single greatest fault in most young players is that they do not take practice seriously enough. If something seems to work for them, they feel as though they've mastered it and don't work on learning new and better ways to do it. Most players work on their strengths, not their weaknesses. This is wrong. Young players see older players doing something in games and they think they

Scrimmage game early in my career. The ball has just been popped right out of my shooting hands.

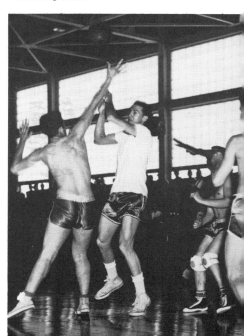

can go right out and do the same thing. They want to
take shortcuts. They don't realize that nothing becomes
perfected without practice.

You start, usually, playing alone, perhaps just shooting. Then, maybe a friend or two joins you. You get up
pickup games. Perhaps you join a kids' team and play in
a local league. You begin to work under coaches. Eventually, you go out for a school team and begin to play in
serious competition. Whether you work out alone or
with others, you should plan what you are going to do
and work at it seriously. Perhaps it is no more complicated than working on a jump-shot. All right, don't just
shoot one or two. Shoot the same shot over and over
again and keep shooting it until you are completely comfortable with it.

I'm not saying you can't have fun. Playing this game,
in practice or in games, is fun. But hold the clowning
down to a minimum. How many baskets can you try to
shoot from behind your back? So you make one. What
good is it? Stay loose, but have a goal and work hard
toward it. Get competitive. See how many of a certain
kind of shot you can make out of twenty attempts.
Then try another twenty and try to make more. Shooting with a buddy, play games like "21" or "horse."

Do you know these games? Probably. In "21" a player picks an area to shoot from. If he makes his shot the
other player must make a shot from the same area. The
first player to make 21 shots wins. In "horse" a player
shoots a certain kind of shot from an area. If he makes it
the other player must make exactly the same kind of
shot from the same area. If he misses he is stuck with the
first letter, h. The first one to be stuck with all five letters loses. Kids, even pro superstars, have been playing
such simple games for years. They're competitive. A
fellow likes to win.

There are a lot of skills a player can practice alone.
Basically, I learned to shoot working out all by myself

on a neighbor's hoop, long hours, day after day, in summer and winter, in sun and rain and snow, often until
after darkness, often until I was late for supper and my
mother was mad at me. I was a bit of a loner as a boy,
and basketball was a blessing to me. And as I look back I
really believe the shooting I do now against the greatest
players in the game—in big arenas, before great crowds,
before writers and broadcasters, with television cameras
following me—was learned when I was a young boy.

A player can practice dribbling alone. He can practice
passing to targets chalked on walls. He can practice
jumping. Pick a wall with some markings on it or get a
ladder and put some markings on it. Crouch and jump,
reaching as high as you can, noting how high you reach.
Then crouch and try to jump higher. You will be surprised how work will increase your jumping ability. Practice rebounding your own shots. Practice fast starts and
stops in balance.

With a pal, play shooting games. Practice eluding him
on your dribbling and on your shooting. And practice
defending him on your dribbling and shooting. Play
one-on-one. One-on-one is about the hardest game ever
invented. The amount of sheer hard work you do trying
to evade and keep up with another fellow play after play
is totally exhausting.

Pros love one-on-one. They're always playing it or
dreaming up possibilities. Rod Hundley used to say Elgin
Baylor was the greatest one-on-one player in the world,
and he wanted to take him on tour, taking on the greatest players in the country before sellout crowds. In his
prime, Elg would have been hard to top. But could he
have beaten Wilt Chamberlain? With Wilt's size and
strength, I'm not so sure. I think Connie Hawkins, Rick
Barry, Oscar Robertson, Earl Monroe, Pete Maravich,
John Havlicek, and Dave Bing would be tough one-on-
one with anyone of reasonably similar size. A big man,
Bob Lanier, won the NBA's one-on-one TV contest in

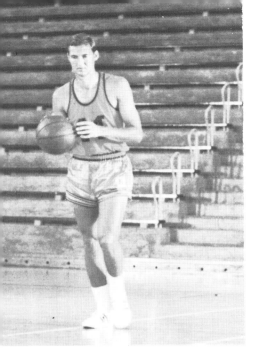 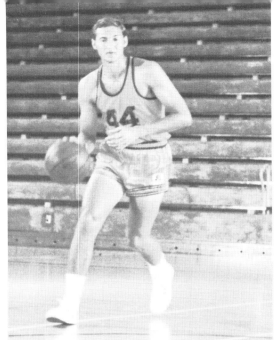

Practicing my jump-shot, I dribble to the
line, brake, make a quick release, and follow-through (next page). Unguarded, I'm
not really making a jump but am working
on a stop in balance and a quick release.
(William Eastabrook for Sunkist Growers)

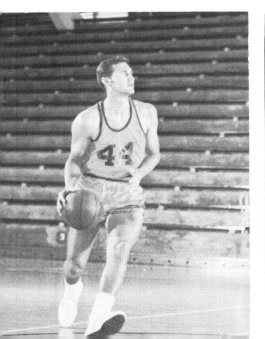 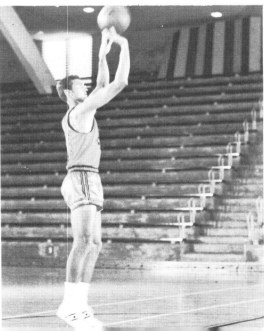

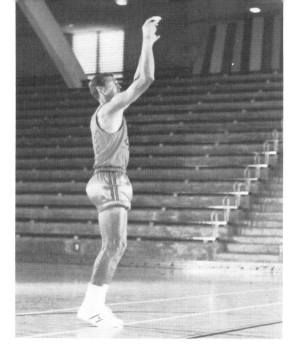

1972, but most of the top players in the league did not enter.

You move up to two-on-two and three-on-three, eventually to full teams. It is in organized competition that you first really learn to play with teammates, to adjust your style to theirs, to make some sacrifices to help them and thus the team.

It is in organized competition that you first learn to play under a coach. You're not going to like everything he does. You may not even like him. You may not think he likes you. But, hopefully your coaches will be men you admire. But it will help if you start with a good attitude.

Accept the fact that the coach is the man in charge. We don't get to pick our generals in battle and we don't get to pick our coaches in games. Whatever he teaches, whether you think he is right or wrong, you will do better and your team will win more games if you do it his way, pulling together, than if everyone goes off doing things his own way.

Most coaches can teach most players something.

Many can teach us many things. Listen. Try. If you want
to go off on your own, turn to individual sports instead
of team sports. Try track or tennis or golf. And even in
these you will find you can benefit by coaching. Basketball is a team game. Practice to play your part as best
you can.

Learn the fundamentals of every aspect of play until
all the moves come automatic to you, until you are comfortable with them and confident of doing them well. It
is all practice and repetition, muscle learning, grooving
of skills. Learn the fundamentals, and you can adjust to
the style of any team you join anywhere. Often in All-
Star games, players must play together with little or no
practice time together. But they know the basics, so
they can fit in with the other players, although not as
well as with their own teams.

In any given game you may have only a few shots, a
few fast-breaks, a few this and a few that. You can't
count on repeating the basic skills in games alone enough
to master them. You must practice repetitiously. Over a
period of practices, work on everything, but generally
emphasize the things you do less well. The things that
are difficult for you to do require more work than the
things that come easier to you.

Practice everything. Gain versatility. You cannot
know how you will mature and what situations you will
find yourself in. You may have to shift positions and
responsibilities. Be prepared. It will get you a starting
spot sometimes when you otherwise would be on the
bench. It may even keep you on a team. Your aim
should always be to improve.

The fellow who is satisfied with himself is overrating
himself. I am never satisfied. I am serious. Others rate
me more highly than I rate myself. I am not being over-
modest. But I am always aware that something could
have been done better.

I have some pet theories about practice. For instance,

I think that as much as possible players should practice at the same times as they play games. They seldom do. We play games at eight at night and practice at ten in the morning or one in the afternoon. Yet I don't know a player who doesn't agree that it is helpful to get into a groove, to do the same things at the same time every day. When you're playing a pro schedule of 100 or so games a season, counting exhibitions and playoffs, it's hard to stay in stride if you don't have a comfortable and familiar routine. My fellow players will blow their tops at this. They wouldn't want their precious nights off taken from them. And I don't blame them. But I honestly think it would help our basketball.

I also believe practices are seldom as organized as they should be. Even on the pro level, there is a lot of talking and clowning around and a lot of wondering what you're accomplishing. This is not true with all coaches, of course. With Fred Schaus, we always felt properly prepared. Bill Sharman is a stickler for details. He basically believes in day-of-the-game practices and meetings. Not just sometimes, but all times. He believes in building a routine you follow forever.

A lot of players resent day-of-the-game practices and meetings. They want to save themselves for the games. I understand this. As you get older you want to conserve energy. But Bill's theory is that you have to get your mind on the game at hand, you have to get physically loose, have to groove your moves the way a fellow rehearses for a speech he has to give at night, and there is much merit to this. However, he doesn't believe in hard practices or long meetings on game days.

I expect different things from coaches on different levels. On the youngest, lowest level, the coach has to be warm and understanding and sympathetic. He has to understand that he is dealing with growing boys who are learning to do things that are difficult for them, things they may not be physically ready to perfect or mentally

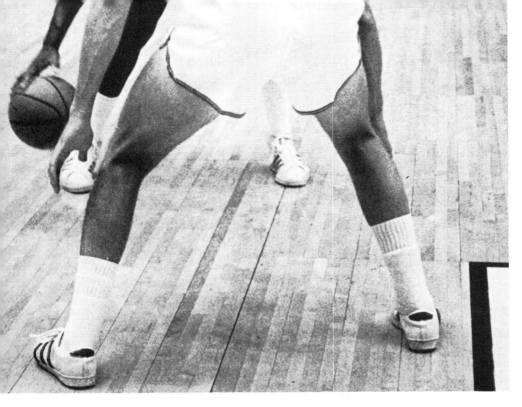

Practicing defense, one-on-one, my footwork is shown as I shuffle to follow the ball
as it is dribbled. I do not cross my feet.
(Photography, Inc.)

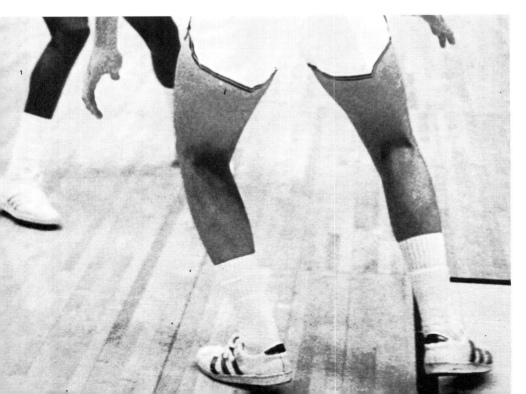

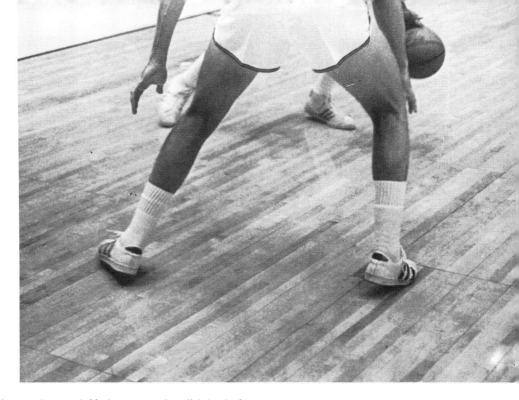

prepared to understand. He has to teach solid, basic fundamentals and give boys time and room to grow and
change. Getting boys into games should be more important to him than winning. Everyone should play. Everyone should try to win, but everyone should play.

As you go higher the coach must be more selective
and demanding. It shouldn't be so on the high school
level, but in many situations coaches have to win to keep
their jobs, so the pressure begins to build early. Also,
college scholarships for many boys depend on their play
on this level, so what should be a fun thing stressing
participation becomes a high-pressure thing stressing
production. This becomes even truer on the college level,
and by the professional level it is, of course, big business.
By then the player who has gotten this far usually has a
wife and children to support and has committed a lot of
his future and maybe his life to the game. Those who are
not going to stay in basketball forever are still giving up
maybe the best years of their lives, say, from ages twenty to thirty, to the sport.

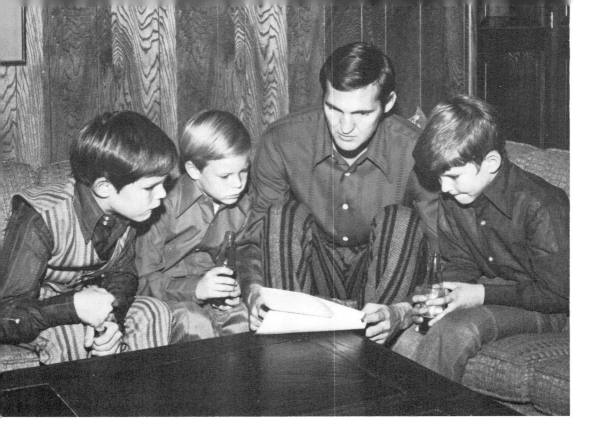

Learning a play, planning a practice, my sons and I sip soft-drinks in our den after dinner. That's David, Mark, Dad, and Michael, left to right. (Photography, Inc.)

The further he goes the more serious the player must become, but he should be aware from the beginning that he is going to be building on a base, and if the base isn't solid, whatever he builds is going to be shaky. And the player should be aware of the pressures on the coach. Mainly, I expect a coach to be a hard worker who asks all his players to work hard, who does not make exceptions, who is fair, and who always means what he says.

It is very important that practices be well-organized, that there be a sense of purpose about them, and the time used well. This is true on any level. It is true even if you are practicing on your own. You should say to yourself, "I am going to work out at least so long today on this."

As you advance into group practice with someone leading it, I think you should play it out. You don't need long practices. Sixty to ninety minutes should be enough. Two hours is a very long practice and is perhaps advisable only before the season begins, when you are building up conditioning.

It is more advisable to use the time you take wisely than to use a lot of time. If you are going to have a one-hour practice you can start by shooting individually for five minutes, then go on to other things.

Basically, you should go from individual practice to small-group practice—one-on-one, two-on-two, and so forth, and drills—and close out the regular practice period with scrimmages. You should loosen up with some calisthenics and light running before practice and close with some lap-running after practice. The younger you are the less you need to loosen up, it seems, but it doesn't hurt to get your muscles warm and loose, to break a sweat before beginning hard work. And it guards against pulled muscles and premature fatigue.

You shouldn't plan your practice schedules too far in advance but should keep them up to date by revising them to suit your immediate needs. You should work on the things you are not doing so well and the things you are going to have to do well to win your next game. It is a cliché, but you should never look too far ahead and should take your schedule one game at a time. The thing you are doing right now is the most important thing in your life. What happened before is gone, and you never know what's going to happen next.

Especially on the lower levels, the players and the coach, if there is one, should go over the rules a little at each session, and the players should quiz one another or be quizzed, because the rules are tools you work with, and it's a terrible handicap not to know what you can and can't do. The objectives of the practice should be explained and discussed briefly, and if there is a game coming up, the game plan, the strategy, discussed. Once the practice begins on the lower levels, the fundamentals should be stressed. If something is done wrong, even if it

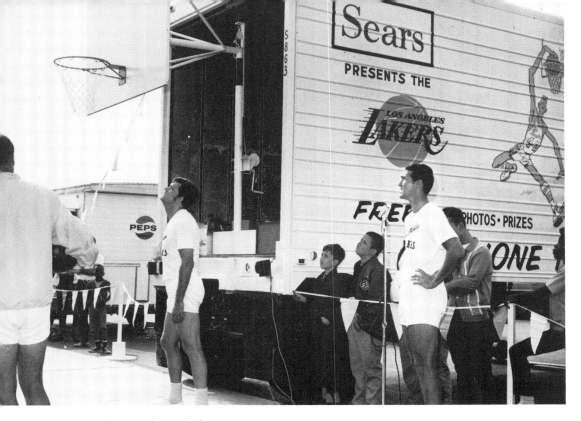

Here I take part in one of the clinics Sears
sponsors with the Lakers. (Sears)

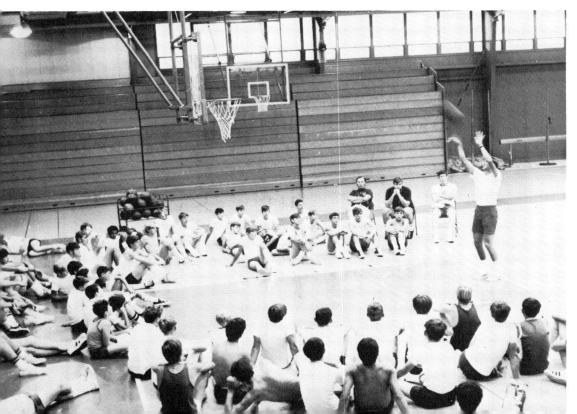

works, the play should be stopped and the basics discussed and the thing run again and again until it is right. There should be no fooling around. That doesn't mean the players can't be loose. But practice is work-time for improvement, it should be spent with a purpose in mind.

The best calisthenics are stretch drills, then short starts and stops, then short sprints. Perhaps some waist-bends and pushups and running in place. Then passing the ball around to get the feel of it, in small circles or rows, not unlike the Harlem Globetrotter drills, but with considerably less clowning.

If a youngster has an injury of any seriousness at all, I suggest he sit it out. Kids shouldn't force themselves or be forced to play. They're not on the pro level, playing for pay, their teammates dependent on them for a living. Youngsters have their whole careers ahead of them. Kids shouldn't goof off or play sick, but they should be realistic about any sickness or injury they have.

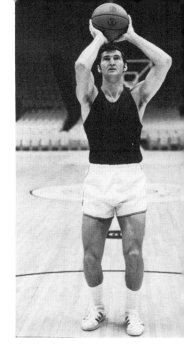

My two-hand overhand set-shooting form. (Photography, Inc.)

Usually, it is best to start with shooting practice. It loosens players up and they enjoy it, and it is, of course, very important. There are many things you can do, and you can vary the things you do and the order you do them from practice to practice to provide variety. Everyone should shoot ten to a hundred free-throws every day. Not everyone has to start with this. The players can take turns. But everyone should get his share in before the workout is over. It is good to use retrievers here as in other shooting practice. The players can take turns serving as retrievers and passing the ball back out to the shooters.

Beyond free-throws, the players should shoot all their other shots, shooting more of those they don't shoot so well. I know it's nice to see that ball go in the basket, but the point is to get a variety of shots in it. You should start in close and gradually work your way out to longer and longer shots, perhaps stretching your range a

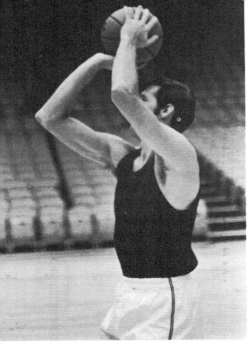

My one-hand shooting style as I practice free-throws. The ball is held steady, on the pads of my hand, elbow aimed at the bucket, and the follow-through is with a limp wrist and a hand waving at the hoop. (Photography, Inc.)

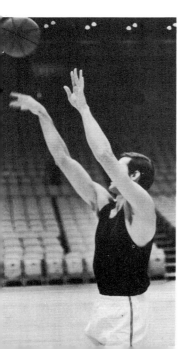

bit. You should shoot from different parts of the court. We all have favorite spots we try to reach, but I don't think the player should limit himself. You can't always choose.

As you practice, begin to shoot as though under game conditions. Pretend there is a man on you and use the fakes you will use, and jump quickly and release quickly as though defensed. There is one special practice I used a lot when I was developing, and that was to have a coach or another player throw me the ball in different places, from where I'd shoot right there and right then, wherever and however I caught the ball. This builds up your quickness, your versatility, your sense of where the basket is.

You should try shots, especially in-close shots, with each hand, just as you should dribble with both hands. One thing that may help here is to try eating with the other hand, opening doors with the other hand, writing with the other hand, doing many things with the other hand to build up your dexterity with it. You don't want to ruin your social graces or your schoolwork, but it's something for spare-time practice.

One shooting trick I never used, but which others have tried with some success was to rig a wire hanger or other sturdy wire inside the rim to reduce its diameter from 18 inches to 16 or 14 inches. It is surprising how big the basket seems when you then start shooting at a normal rim. This is a fun thing you may want to fool around with. But it is not good to discourage players by making shooting even more difficult than it is.

If something isn't working for you, stop and try to figure out why or ask a coach or an experienced player to watch you so he may be able to tell you what you are doing wrong.

It is nice to be helpful, especially when asked, but too much instruction has ruined many players, and the fact

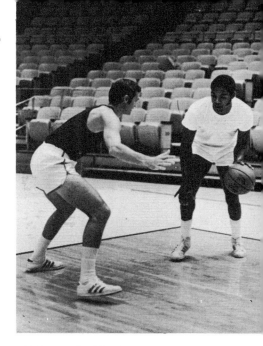

is that few players, especially young ones, understand the fundamentals well enough to teach. Anyway, everyone develops his own style.

If a player is having trouble he can usually find a coach or an experienced player, perhaps at a clinic, who can help him. I give clinics for the Lakers and for Sears and have made instructional films for Sunkist Growers. In practice you should shoot very well, better than in games. For some players it's very hard when they get on the court when it counts.

Shoot a jump-shot. Then fake a jump-shot and drive. Shoot from the corners. Shoot from outside. The thing is to become as good as you possibly can. And you never know how much better you will become as you mature. The fellow who shoots 100 jump-shots has a better chance to become a good jump-shooter than the one who shoots ten. Don't play to exhaustion. But build up endurance.

Defensing Jim McMillian man-to-man in practice, I keep one hand "on the ball," shifting from a medium right hand to a low left hand as his dribble moves the ball around. (Photography, Inc.)

Pair up and work on one-on-one some. Put a defense against an offense. Start loose and tighten up. Play some of the games we have discussed, "21" and "horse." Or "round the world," in which the players start in one corner and gradually work their way in a semicircle beyond the free-throw line to the other corner, taking about seven shots side-to-side, then working their way back, taking turns, the first to sink 21 winning.

Work with a teammate on tips and rebounds. Try to keep the ball in play by tapping it back and forth off the board.

Line up the players you have in two rows and run layup practice. A player in row A dribbles up and lays the ball in, then goes to the end of row B. The first player in row B takes A's layup and passes it to the next player breaking off row A and goes to the end of row A, and so forth. You've all seen it. It is good practice and you should try first from one side, then from straight

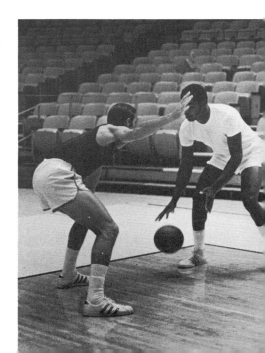

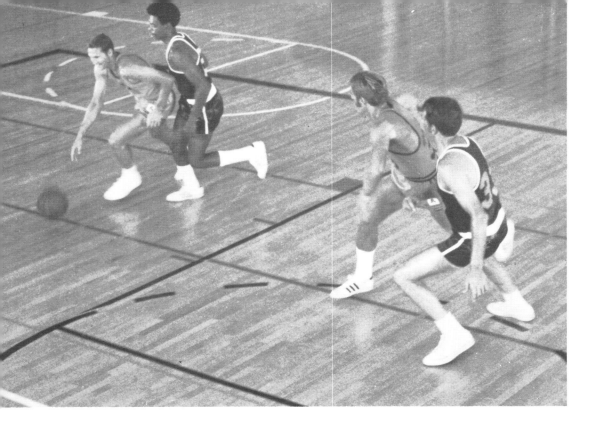

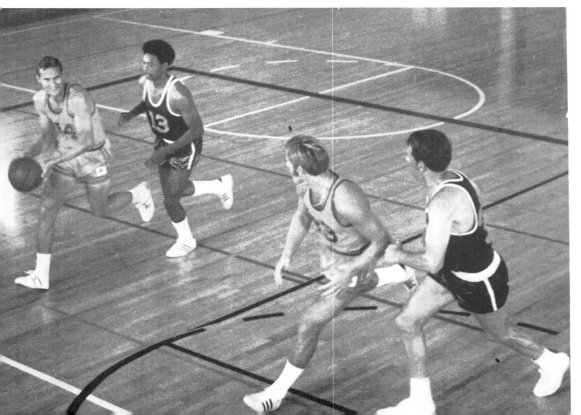

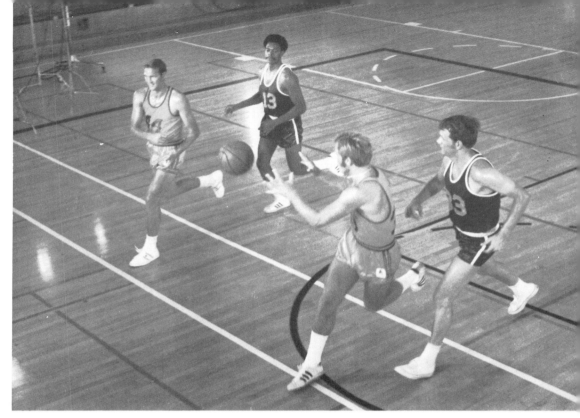

down the middle, then from the other side, right- and left-handed. See how many you can put in without a miss. The same drill can be run culminating in jump-shots from the free-throw line.

Divide the players into two rows. Let two players from each row dribble and pass the ball the length of the court or from midcourt into a layup. Try to get down a whole row without a miss. The row that misses has to start all over again after the whole row has shot. From the far end of the court this is a good fast-break drill. Work it with two men, then three men. Then work it with defenders, two attackers on one, two-on-two, three-on-two, three-on-three. This is a defensive drill, too, of course.

Basically, a man, presumably a rebounder, takes the ball at one end and fires an outlet pass to a teammate to get the break going. Usually, the first man to break will do so down the middle and the pass will go to the mid-

Happily heading out on a two-man fast-break, I put the ball on the court as I get the jump on Art Williams and Pat Riley busts inside of Rod Hundley (left). Then I pass the ball to Pat (above) and we are well in front, sure of a "sure" shot, cameras turning to preserve this moment for posterity on an instructional film. (William Eastabrook for Sunkist Growers)

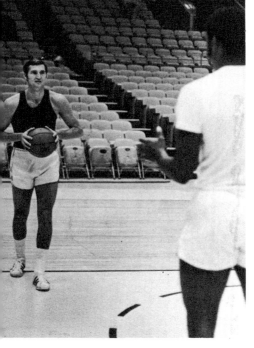

Practicing the direct two-hand pass with Jim McMillian. Actually, I'm holding the ball a bit low to begin with (it should be chest-high) and have made my stride too soon. You tend to get careless after a while and must guard against this. (Photography, Inc.)

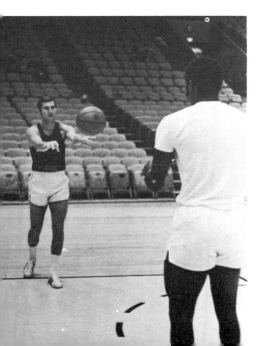

dleman with others involved in the break flanking him. There should be a trailer following and a defender hanging back. Preferably, the best ballhandler will be the middleman. He can work it either of two ways. He can pass back and forth between his flankers as the break sweeps upcourt, or he can dribble and pass to them as they reach drive-in range. Much depends on whether the defense is in position to cover the flankers and intercept passes.

This must be run over and over again. There is no way a fast-break is going to work consistently in games if it has not been grooved in practice. It takes timing to coordinate with teammates in a fast-moving break. And at the end of the break, get up high to put in as sure a lay-up as possible. You can sometimes put chairs or towels around the court to force players to dribble around them. This is similar to some skiing races and builds dexterity and agility.

Work on your dribbling—slow, fast, low, high, with both hands. After a while, work against a single defender, then against two defenders. These are also good defense drills. The defender tries to get the ball away from the dribbler without fouling. Dribble end-to-end with a teammate, periodically passing back and forth. Practice your quick stop off the dribble, maintaining balance, protecting the ball, your feet in the proper position for pivoting.

Work on your passing, all kinds of passes, with one man, with two, in facing rows. Practice passing the football pass to kick off a fast-break, the pass to the pivot, the pass to the man breaking for the basket. Run relay races. If the ball is passed swiftly enough it is possible to run end-to-end legally without a dribble. In passing practice, start with short, soft passes and gradually build up your length and velocity as you move toward drills. Work on the timing, which is critical to a good passing game.

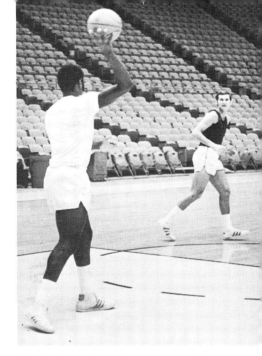

Work on figure-8 weaves. Players can work off a pivot, taking and returning passes as they move in a figure-8 pattern. Or they can work in a simple figure 8, giving and getting passes as they move toward each other and across one another's path. These weaves are critical on offense, anyway, to stimulate movement into a stagnant attack and to freeze the ball.

Players can perfect passing in small groups. For example, two can alternate passes to one receiver. As soon as he gets the ball he should return it to one or the other. The one who gets it can return it right back to him. You can step up the speed gradually, building up not only your passing but receiving. Don't just get rid of the ball. Use sound passes. If the two gradually spread out it becomes a good test of the single player's peripheral vision.

Work on out-of-bounds passes and plays, offensively and defensively. This is critical. It should be done systematically, but it can be done carelessly. The passer must know where his potential receivers are going, the receivers must know where to go. Different plays may be developed for different situations, such as out-of-bounds play from your own end, from the sidecourt, and from under the basket you are attacking. A few possible plays are illustrated in this chapter.

The fast-break football pass practiced by Jim McMillian and me. (Photography, Inc.)

Even if you have a team that does not use a lot of set plays, you must have some out-of-bounds plays you can execute quickly and reliably. You do not need many, but you need a few for variety, and everyone must know his assignment. The first aim is to get the ball to a teammate. The second aim—unless the situation makes it the first consideration—is to set up a swift move at the basket. You must build in safety factors. If you are trying for a shooter you must have a secondary receiver available. In any case, you must have a man to protect on defense in case of a steal.

The man taking the ball in-bounds must call out the play, by number or color. He should be at arm's length

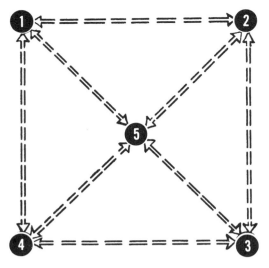

SQUARE

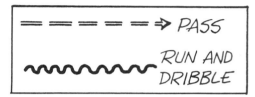

= = = = = = → PASS

〜〜〜〜〜〜 RUN AND DRIBBLE

PASSING DRILLS

Here are three basic passing drills. The square and the lane should be self-explanatory. The single-file drill goes as follows: As 3 and 4 pass each other, 3 passes to 4 and goes to far end of the opposite line. 2 slants out as 4 passes to 2 and goes to his opposite end, while 2 goes on to meet 5, etc.

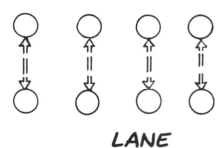

LANE

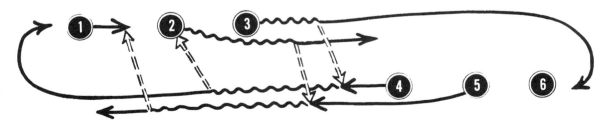

SINGLE FILE

from the sideline so the defender cannot harass him un-
reasonably. And he should get the play going by a shout
or by slapping the ball. Line up two or three players
horizontally or vertically and at the signal break them in
one direction or another. Since the defense cannot know
which way they are going and when, the split-second
advantage the offense has in this case should be sufficient to free a receiver if the pass is made quickly and
crisply.

If the defense is protecting effectively, it is sometimes
good to throw high passes to your taller players, which
are more difficult to defend against. Often it is good to
feed a quick return pass to the original passer as he
breaks inbounds, as he will often be uncovered the moment after he releases the ball and can cut for the basket
sharply.

If time is running out and you need the basket badly,
pass to your best shooter, unless he is covered too closely. Perhaps pass to your best ballhandler or the man least
likely to be defended and let him set up a screen that
allows your good shooters to cut him off for passes. The

Teaching the circle routine for practice passing by the hoop hung on the garage of my
home, I work with, left to right, sons David
and Michael, Kevin Hawkins, and son Mark.
(Photography, Inc.)

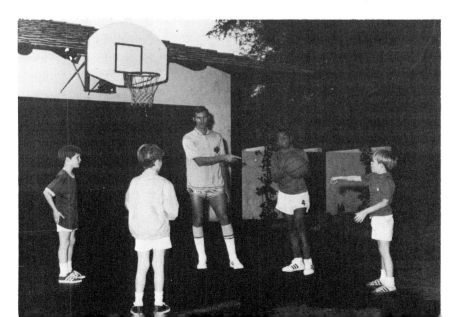

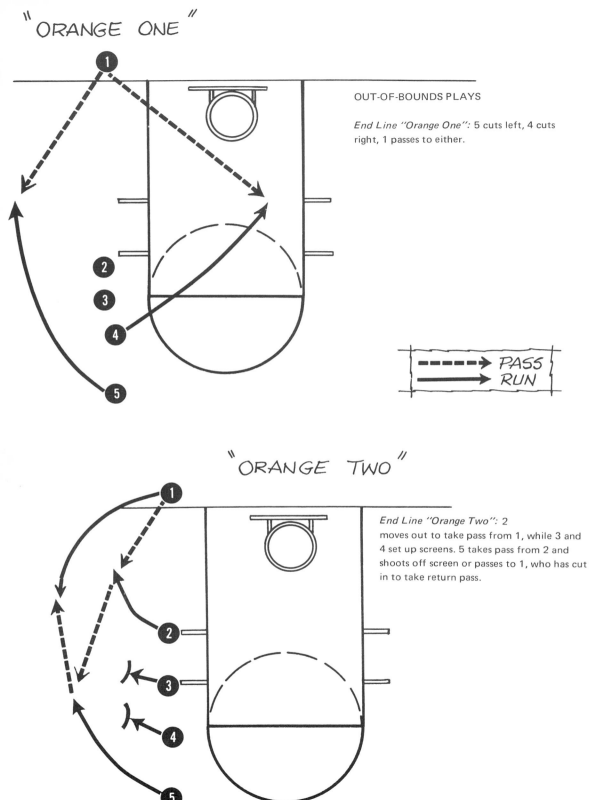

"ORANGE ONE"

OUT-OF-BOUNDS PLAYS

End Line "Orange One": 5 cuts left, 4 cuts right, 1 passes to either.

PASS
RUN

"ORANGE TWO"

End Line "Orange Two": 2 moves out to take pass from 1, while 3 and 4 set up screens. 5 takes pass from 2 and shoots off screen or passes to 1, who has cut in to take return pass.

"PURPLE ONE"

End Line "Purple One": 5 cuts off to left, 2 crosses out to right, 3 and 4 move to right side to set up screens. 1 passes to 2 for screened shot or to 5 if open. 1's pass to 5 should be just ahead of screeners.

PASS

RUN

"PURPLE TWO"

End Line "Purple Two": 3 and 4 hold position. 5 cuts off to left, 2 crosses out to right, but immediately doubles back behind 3 and 4, who have faked move inside and remained to screen. 1 passes to 2 or 5 for shot.

"WHITE ONE"

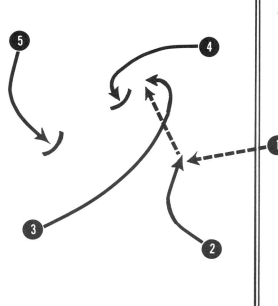

Sidelines "White One": 2 cuts to take pass from 1 as 4 and 5 set screens. 3 cuts behind to take pass from 2.

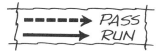

PASS
RUN

"WHITE TWO"

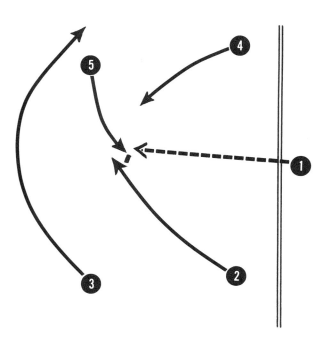

Sidelines "White Two": 5 breaks into high post and takes pass from 1, while 3 cuts wide outside circle. 2 cuts in front of 5 and 5 hands off to 2 or turns and passes underneath to 3.

less time you have left the less elaborate the play can be. Sometimes the high pass to the pivot is fastest, and so best. But if he is closely guarded the good outside shot may be preferable. Try to get the ball to any player who can get free in his best shooting area.

Work these plays without your good defenders knowing what is coming up as a defensive drill. Stress shutting off the best shooters, whether the initial pass is to them or not, and stress a tight defense in close to the basket, forcing the other side to take their desperation shot from as far out as possible. Always position a good rebounder in close to the hoop to protect against the fast follow-up shot.

Build up a book of as many set plays as you want to use and practice them repetitiously until you are completely comfortable with them. As I have said, I don't believe in using too many set plays, but I believe every team must have some to meet various situations. You can copy or develop your own, but some are diagrammed herein for your use. Plays should be tailored to a team's strength and a foe's weakness. They should be designed to free a player for the easiest shot possible and to give the ball to your best shooters in their best places.

Set plays restrict a team, and used too often they can be recognized and defensed, but they are extremely handy tools and tend to discipline a team.

Vary signals so that the defensive players cannot anticipate which play is coming up. Perhaps the defense will recognize it rapidly, but this will simply serve to make the offensive task more difficult, which is useful. Run crisply, a sound play should still succeed.

Almost all offensive drills turn into defensive drills, too. Spend as much time on defense as you do on offense, perhaps more if you need it. Don't break up your regular lineup any more than necessary. Keep your starting five intact as much as possible, but work in the subs who will have to work with them in games. Put your starters on defense as often as on offense.

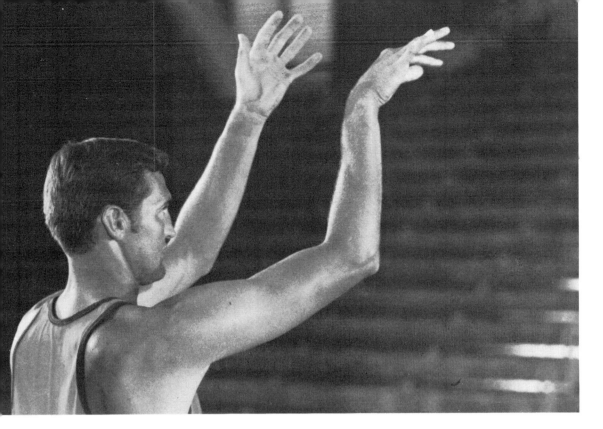

Following through on the finish of a one-hander, I have practiced my shooting for some 25 years now and I'll probably go on practicing even after I retire. Practice may be hard sometimes, but shooting is fun. (William Eastabrook for Sunkist Growers)

When a play stalls or doesn't work, don't just cut it off but flow back into your normal pattern. A play will not work all the time. Don't let it discourage or disconcert you. Carry on with your usual offense. But a set play should work a high percentage of the time—perhaps six out of ten times if used sparingly—or there is no point to it. It must be practiced until run efficiently. When it isn't working, don't force it. If you see it is beaten, flow back into your regular attack.

The plays in this chapter are good, basic ones, but they do not take into account the skills of the personnel on your team. Diagram plays to stress your strengths. Keep them uncomplicated. You will get more results from sound execution of a simple play than erratic execution of a difficult play. It is the old Green Bay Packer system.

Do not overdo scrimmages. Run short but intense ones. Do not leave your game in the gym, but prepare for the game in the gym. As often as possible, use a full court and referees, follow the rules, simulate game action. Scrimmage free for a while, then scrimmage on special situations. Set up a situation where your team is "X number" of points behind and must press for the ball and shoot rapidly. Set up a situation where your team is "X number" of points ahead and must stall to kill the clock. Set up a situation where you in-bound for a last basket. Work with and against the various zones. The possibilities are numerous. Stress those that you have not worked well in games.

By putting your starters on defense as well as on offense, it becomes a defensive drill against these crisis situations. As much as possible, keep score. Perhaps you'll want to punish with extra laps after practice the team that permits the most points rather than the team that scores the fewest. It's the same team, obviously, but it's a psychological trick that gets a team to thinking defense. And you're not really punishing anyone severely. It can be fun.

Sometimes pro practices are wars. Remember, you're teammates, not foes.

Practice can be fun, but it must be taken seriously. It has to have a point. And the point is improvement. The most fun of all in basketball is winning.

9. Off the Court

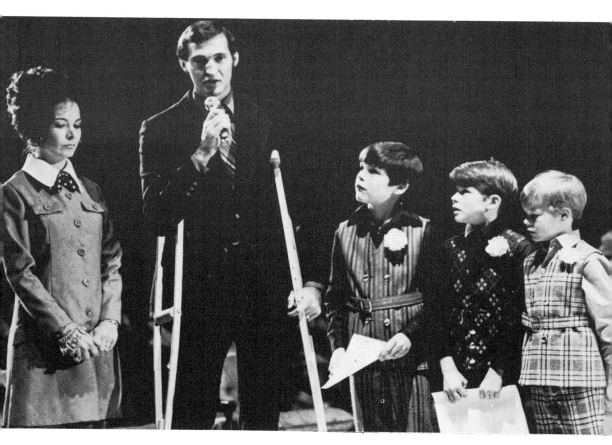

A night honoring me given by the Lakers and southern California fans. Here, on crutches, recovering from my knee operation, mike in hand, I thank everyone, flanked by my wife, Jane, and sons David, Michael, and Mark. (Photography, Inc.)

ON THE SECOND day of March 1971, I was reaching for a ball, trying to break up a fast-break, when I collided with Bob Kauffman, the 6-8, 240-pound center of the Buffalo team, and we went down and he rolled on top of me and the inside of my right knee was torn up. The complicated medical term was that I suffered a torn medial collateral ligament. The fact is that it hurt real bad and scared me a great deal.

I was thirty-two years old, in my eleventh year as a pro, nineteenth year in organized competition, and didn't know how many years I had left in the game. I was having a good season, although I often got very tired, especially after a number of hard games in a row, suffered slumps more severe than before, and sometimes had to force myself to keep going all-out.

Still, I was leading my team in scoring and was second in the league in assists, and in general, was doing a good all-around job as a floor leader. I knew my loss for the season would finish off our playoff chances. Actually, some of the men played inspired ball to make up for my loss, and the team gave a good account of itself in the playoffs, upsetting favored Chicago before falling to the eventual champion, Milwaukee.

I went into the hospital, where an operation was performed by Dr. Robert Kerlan's associate, Dr. Frank Jobe, and I spent time in bed, then time on crutches, before I could take off the cast. I hobbled to and from a lot of games, including one in which the Laker organization and fans gave me a night in my honor, which had been planned before the injury.

I was uncomfortable, though it was a great thrill. I mean inside I am a proud person and it is not every person who has a night in his honor. The money I am paid and the applause I receive really have been ample repayment. I do not believe an athlete who is highly paid should accept gifts. Funds collected on "my night" went into a scholarship fund at West Virginia University.

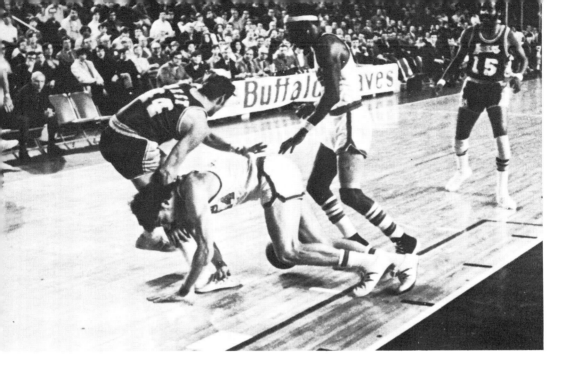

Here's how I got injured late in the 1971 season. I was trying to intercept a pass when the Braves' big Bob Kauffman, 6-8 and 240, crashed into me, bending my right knee the wrong way and tearing it up inside. As I grab my leg in pain, the Braves' Em Bryant continues with the play. (Photos by Robert L. Smith, "Creaking Trees," Elma, N. Y.)

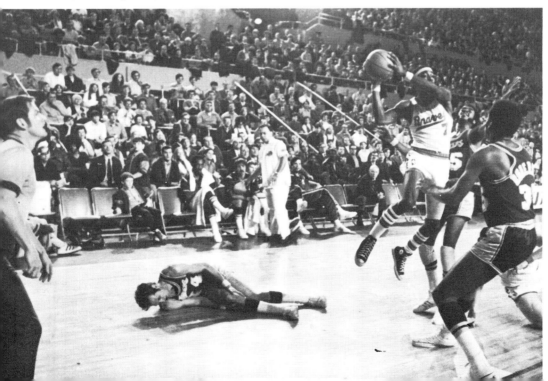

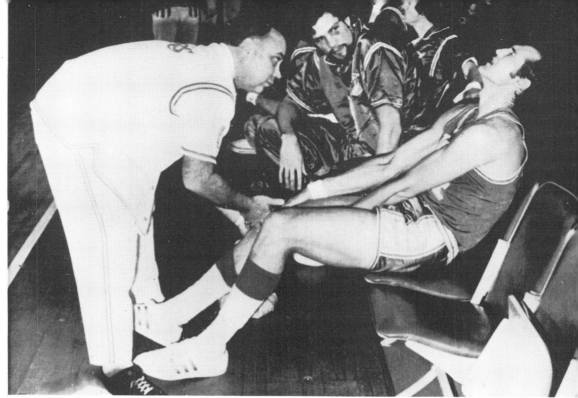

I did not want it to be a farewell. I wanted to go on playing, though I was not sure for how long. At one time I set as goals at least ten years and 20,000 points scored in regular-season play. But after attaining those goals I still wanted to go on playing. I wanted to play on an NBA championship team, but after narrowly missing this honor many times I could not wait for it, but out of a clear sky, it came. I always said I wanted to quit before I fell off in ability and was embarrassing myself, and I hope to stick to that, though it is hard to quit on something you love. You must remember that the average person—worker of any kind—can go on doing what he is doing most of his life. The average athlete who is making a great living must quit young.

I suppose getting hurt the way I did, getting forced out of action, increased my desire to get back into the game. I think this happened to Wilt Chamberlain when he tore up a knee early in the 1969-70 season and was able to come back from his operation and recuperation period before the end of the season. Possibly it hap-

In pain, my knee having just been severely injured, I moan and groan as trainer Frank O'Neill and teammate Fred Hetzel look me over in the top shot. Below, the knee bandaged and packed in ice, I limp off, aided by Hetzel. This was in Buffalo and I was on my way back to L.A., to an operation that sidelined me the rest of the 1970-71 season. (AP Wirephotos)

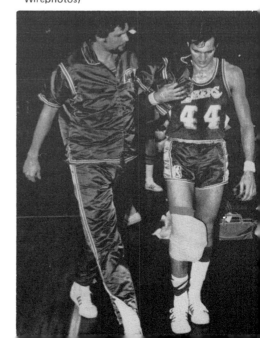

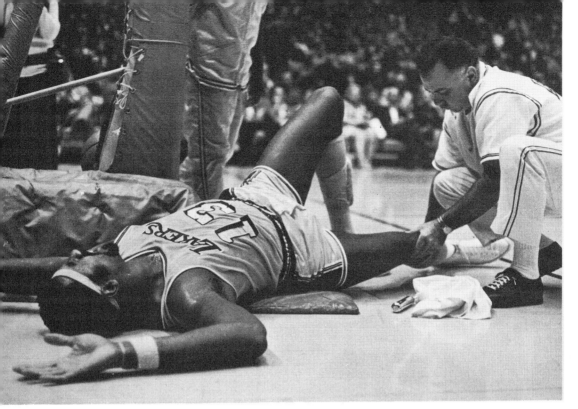

In pain, his knee just having been torn up inside, Wilt Chamberlain lies flat on the Forum court as trainer Frank O'Neill examines him. (Photography, Inc.)

pened to Elgin Baylor when he tore up his knee in the 1965 playoffs. You want to make the decision yourself, not have it forced on you.

In some ways, basketball must be the hardest of games to endure. I mean that. Check the records. The career span of the average basketball pro is less than that of those in baseball, football and hockey. There are many more players aged thirty or more, or thirty-five or more, in baseball, football, and hockey than there are in basketball. I think it's because the bursts of hard running, often prolonged for many minutes at a time, on hardwood courts contributes to it, especially in the legs. When you get to be thirty in basketball, people start expecting you to retire.

You don't get hit the way you do in football or hockey, but there is plenty of body contact. And an athlete's greatest physical assets are his legs, and I think the legs are punished more in basketball than in other games.

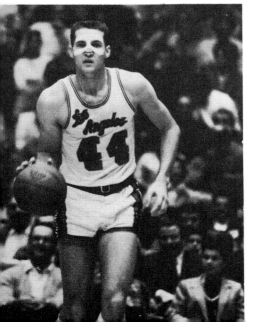

My nose broken for the umpteenth time, bandaged until I look like some sort of Halloween villain, I start upcourt. A broken nose hurts, but you can play with it. (Sports Illustrated photo by Neil Leifer © Time, Inc.)

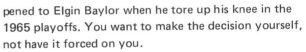

There is a lot of twisting and turning and jumping and coming down on those hard courts, and it tortures your legs and especially your knees. Aside from backs in football, all basketball players seem to suffer more from knee injuries than any other athletes.

I suppose there is a certain amount of wearing down of the muscles and ligaments and joints of the knee, because these injuries become more common the more the player plays and the older he gets. Certainly they are not uncommon, and many players have come back from knee injuries. Elgin Baylor's knee injury was a lot worse than mine. Part of his kneecap was torn off. He suffered severely but made a fairly successful comeback. Wilt made an amazing comeback from his knee operation.

I did the knee-strengthening exercises prescribed for me and worked out hard, and I recovered and resumed playing at my former level. But it does scare you a little, you're so dependent on your knees. Of course, this knee injury was not the only injury I've suffered in basketball, but it was by far the most severe.

It's no secret that I've had more than my share of injuries. My nose has been broken ten times, my hands have been broken twice. I've broken fingers, pulled and torn muscles, twisted and sprained my fingers, my wrists and my ankles, and been bruised from head to toe. I've had my share of sicknesses—from the flu to strep throat. Whenever I could I played. The pro plays in pain. It's the job. You're well-paid for it. I'm not unique.

Sometimes you can't play. I missed 25 games in the 1963 season, 14 games in 1967, 31 games in 1968, 21 games in 1969, 13 games in 1971, and other games in other seasons—146 games in twelve seasons as a professional. Plus some playoff games two seasons. On the other hand I have played virtually the full schedule, 70 or more games, plus preseason and postseason games, seven seasons. I missed only five games in the 1971-72 season.

It annoys me when I'm called injury-prone, though

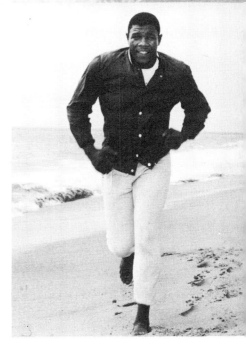

Postoperation workouts: Jim "Bad News" Barnes running (above); Wilt Chamberlain (below) lifting weights with mending leg; also bicycling for real or with stationary mount, as in background. (Photography, Inc.)

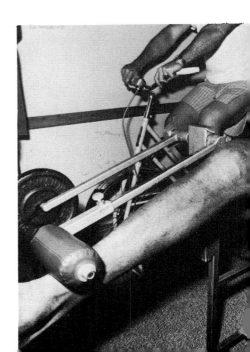

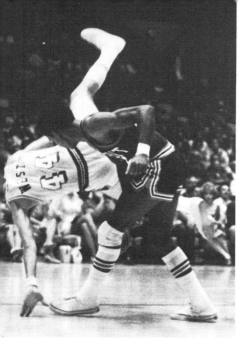

Stopping suddenly, Dave Bing accidentally flipped me over his back and I landed flat on my face. This time I wasn't hurt too bad. (Photography, Inc.)

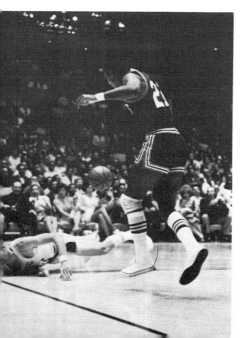

maybe I am. Dr. Kerlan says my muscles are not as elastic as the average player's, and some have said I throw myself around a bit too recklessly on court. Compared to many pros, I appear frail. But at 6-3 I weigh 190 pounds or so, which is, as I have pointed out, heavyweight-boxer weight.

I don't think you can spare yourself. There are certain things you can do to protect against injuries, but beyond that you have to play the game aggressively and take your chances. I might point out that I have played more than 1,000 games since I began my career back in high school.

Few players are going to play long without pulling muscles. If you break your nose, chances are you'll keep getting it broken. This is my specialty. I'll never forget the doctor back in Charleston who set the first and said he hadn't done it right and had to reset it, and did it right then, without an anesthetic, and it hurt so much I almost jumped right off the table. But even when they give you that shot to kill the pain, the needle is painful. Well, it's like going to the dentist. You have to go.

Doctors Kerlan and Jobe and trainer Frank O'Neill keep me patched up, and I go on. I have spoken to them and to others, and I have my own experiences to call on to provide you with some advice in this area.

As you grow up and mature, your physical strength and agility, the toughness of your bones and muscles, will develop. You can help yourself along. Walk and run as much as you can to build up your legs. Off-seasons, turn out for track, or run on your own. Start slowly and build up your speed. Don't strain yourself to the point of pulling muscles, but take short sprints, maybe 20 yards in length. Those are the sort of sprints you'll take in games. And run for distance to build up the strength in your legs, your heart, and the capacity of your lungs.

Build up your hands, arms, and upper body, too. Do

push-ups, pull-ups, sit-ups, and reasonable stretching exercises. Carry around a hard rubber ball, perhaps a tennis ball, to squeeze a lot, strengthening your hands and fingers. Hold a stick in both hands and turn it as far as you can to build up your wrists.

Some weight lifting may help, but this can be dangerous and should be done only under supervision with your goals clearly understood. Some isometrics may help. Clasp your fingers together and pull against yourself. Sit on a chair, grip it, and pull up. Press your hands against a tabletop and press down or against a wall and press in. A lot of muscle can be built in simple, individual ways. If you do weight lift, lift just enough to tax the muscles and then increase the number of repetitions, not the weight.

Riding a bike is excellent exercise. Unless your coach cautions you against it, swimming is all right. It doesn't hurt you in any way, despite the fact that some are against it. A wide variety of muscles are put to use and it tends to loosen you up. In season it should be done in moderation and it will neither hurt you too much nor help you too much. It is just one of many exercises you can use.

There are a number of old-wives' tales, things that have been passed down through the years as fact but actually are far more fancy. One is that exercise takes off weight, adds to height, or hurts digestion. Another is that weight lifting and swimming are always harmful. Exercise is helpful in reducing when done in conjunction with diets, but the only real way to lose weight is to cut down on the calories. A 155-pound person would have to walk around 140 miles, run 15 miles or do 5,000 push-ups to lose a single pound, I am told.

Some young fellows want to add weight. To do so, build up the sugars, starches, and fats in your meals and drink a couple of malted milks a day. Mainly, unless you

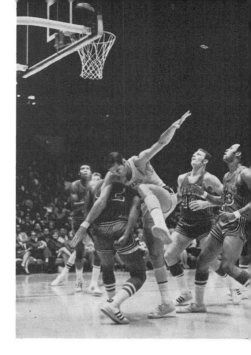

Like a big plane coming down for a landing, I have just shot and have my wings outspread as I glide through three foes, Walt Hazzard, John Vallely, and Lou Hudson. Or is "crash" a better word than "glide"? (Photography, Inc.)

In full-flight again, wings outspread, I slam past Bill Bridges en-route to another crash-landing. (Photography, Inc.)

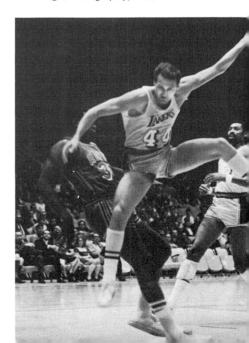

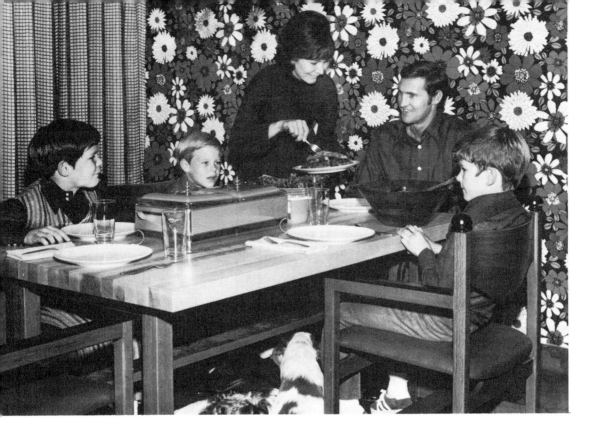

Dinnertime in the dinette of the West household shows Jane serving her men—David, Mark, Jerry, and Michael—plus a waiting dog beneath the table. (Photography, Inc.)

have a special weight problem that needs a doctor's advice, good exercise and the proper diet will keep you trim. I believe diet and rest are the two most important factors in staying fit, especially in young people. I don't believe you have any idea how much energy you are expending playing hard games.

The best things to eat for a balanced diet are a lot of lean meat, fish, fruit, vegetables, whole-grain items, and milk. Dr. Kerlan simply says to get your share of proteins, carbohydrates, and fats. He's not much of one for fad diets or a lot of food supplements, such as vitamin pills. He feels that if you eat right the food will provide the right vitamins. If you don't, you may need some vitamin supplements, such as Vitamin C, currently recommended to combat colds.

Have some juice or fruit for breakfast, some cooked or dry cereal, some toast with butter or honey, some milk or cocoa. Sometimes have eggs, but avoid too many

fried eggs or fried bacon or other fried foods. Go for
fruit, soup, meat (such as steak, roast beef, lamb chops,
liver), fish, or a macaroni-type dish, a green vegetable, a
piece of bread, ice cream, and milk for lunch. For supper, try soup, meat, or fish, maybe a baked potato, a
vegetable or salad, a light dessert like Jello and milk or
tea.

On game days, eat three to four hours before the
game. It takes about three hours to digest the average
meal. A stroll after this meal will aid your digestion. You
play better and sleep better on an empty stomach. Although I've known players who could eat hot dogs or
pizzas before games and perform well, they are the
exceptions.

I favor a small steak, a baked potato, tea, and maybe
a piece of chocolate four to six hours before a game. If
you suffer from hunger-pangs eating this long before a
game, try a can of Metrecal or some such thing an hour
or so before you have to play.

I avoid spicy foods most of the time, and especially
on game days. I'm not saying you can't ever have spa-
ghetti or a pizza or a hamburger smothered in onions or
a hot dog, but pick your time carefully.

Actually, carbohydrates are the most rapidly di-
gested, so cereals, unfried potatoes, macaroni dishes,
peas, beans, corn, beets, and sugar foods such as sugar or
honey to stir into your tea, and a chocolate bar for
quick energy are good prior to games. Milk fills the
body's needs for calcium, but it is heavy and hard to
digest and should be drunk slowly and never taken in the
pregame meal.

After your digestive walk, don't be afraid to lay
down. In any event, relax. It is an old-wive's tale that
people should not rest after eating. A player needs his
rest. And the younger he is the more he needs it. Young
players often need up to ten hours sleep a night. Later
on this may be cut to eight. I take a nap early in the
afternoon on game days. So do most athletes, I believe.

Some can't. But do it early enough so you won't be still half-asleep by gametime.

One of the problems is that most persons get up in the morning and go to work when they are fresh, where many athletes get up many hours before their games and may be tired from a long day by gametime. Thus seek some rest at least an hour before you go to the game, even if it's only sitting down and getting off your feet. Avoid reading or watching television or other things that may tire your eyes just before going to games.

Don't be afraid to shower before games, just don't stay under the water too long. Often, a short shower will refresh you. Some players grab a quick refreshing shower at halftimes. Some such as Wilt often change to clean, dry uniforms.

It's another old-wives' tale that drinking water is harmful during games, but a lot of ice-water that is put away fast and not sipped might hurt. Mainly, rinse your mouth out or, better yet, chew gum. If you're playing under hot conditions, salt food freely and possibly take some salt tablets between games.

I may sip a little soft-drink or chew lemons and or-anges at halftime. I don't want to be bloated. After a game I won't eat or drink right away. I try to unwind. Usually, you're emotionally high and physically low. Take your time. Gather yourself. If you're going to go to bed right away, don't eat much more than soup, a small sandwich, maybe hot chocolate, milk, or a milk-shake. If you're going to stay up awhile, you can eat a bit more. An hour or two after a game I'll sometimes have a steak.

I get wound up pretty tight and get a nervous stom-ach before games. And I'm still pretty well-coiled after games. It's my way, but I don't recommend it. If you're looser, fine. There's nothing wrong with going out and unwinding after games. Everyone is entitled to a little fun in life. Just keep it within reason. If basketball means something to you, don't abuse your body.

When you're old enough a little beer may not hurt you. I said a little. I don't really know what hard liquor does for anyone. It's clear by now that smoking is something close to suicidal. So are most drugs and pills. I'm not going to lecture you. It's your life. Use your head. It takes more guts to walk away from trouble than it does to do what some are doing. Anyone who pops pills, smokes pot, or indulges in anything like that is stupid. Why take in poison? Be your own man. Lead your own life. Wisely.

Although I don't think it will hurt you to loosen up before games, Dr. Kerlan says that unless you are sick or stiff or sore, the younger you are the less of this you need. For the most part the usual shooting practice on court just before games will loosen you sufficiently, but a little stretching and running in place may help, too.

Make sure you've got good equipment on. This includes good shoes and sweatsocks that fit, an athletic supporter and a uniform that fits. If you have injuries that have to be bandaged, make sure they are bandaged. It's a funny thing, but most players don't know why they do or don't tape their ankles. They just started doing it or they never started doing it, and that's it. However, most players who have had a sprained ankle tape their ankles forever after for games, and they should. Once they have been weakened, they must be protected.

Dr. Kerlan and the Lakers feel very strongly about taping ankles. A fellow who has sprained an untaped ankle is subject to a $50 fine. Yet, some don't tape their ankles. You know who one is? That's right, me. But I've never had a sprained ankle. It's more comfortable to play without tape, and apparently I have strong ankles. However, it is an old-wives tale, according to Dr. Kerlan, that taped ankles lead to knee injuries. The theory here is that if your ankle won't give under pressure, your knee will.

In any event, it does no good to tape your ankle un-

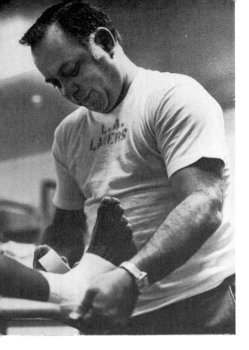

Taping an ankle properly, using a sort of figure-8 system, Frank O'Neill prepares Jim McMillian's leg for a workout. It is no good and perhaps even risky simply to tape an ankle. Those who wish to do it should go to a trainer or athletic doctor and learn the right way. (Photography, Inc.)

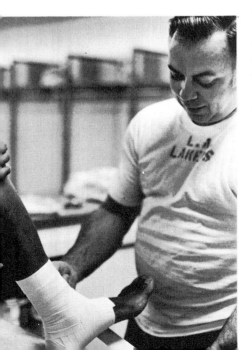

less you tape it properly. In this chapter there are pictures showing our trainer, Frank O'Neill, taping Jim McMillian's ankle properly. If you don't have a trainer or a coach who knows how to do it right, go to a trainer or a coach or a doctor who does, and learn. It's simple enough.

Usually, it helps to spray on a skin-toughener first, because constant taping and untaping of ankles before and after games may prove very irritating. There is a sort of "under-gauze" that helps. O'Neill says he considers ankle-taping excellent preventive medicine. Neither he nor Dr. Kerlan advise taping or bracing knees unless an injury makes it necessary. Nor is O'Neill a great believer in a lot of rubdowns, though he will give them where an athlete feels he needs them. He does believe in loosening up and stretching before games.

Let's look at some of the injuries the athlete may have to deal with, with or without a coach or trainer to handle them. The more severe they seem the more likely that a doctor should be seen. If in doubt, go to a doctor. Treat your ailments yourself only when they are simple, and a skilled person is not available to help you.

Foot blisters come mainly from improperly fitted shoes and socks. Sterilize the area of the blister, puncture with a sterile needle, press the fluid out gently, remove excess dead skin carefully, cover with a medicated cream and bandage with sterile gauze and tape. Change this bandage daily until the blister has healed. Calluses (hard, thick skin formations) can be filed down by a trainer or a doctor but should not be cut except by an expert.

If you twist or sprain your ankle, get off it, soak it in a tub of ice water, or apply ice compresses to it for a half-hour to avoid swelling. Avoid heat treatments, wrap it tightly with an elastic bandage, and stay off it as much as possible for 14 hours or longer until the pain lessens.

If you twist or sprain your knee, use ice for 20 to 30

minutes and then rest it as much as possible for 14 hours
or more. In this case you can apply some moist heat 15
to 20 minutes before resuming use of it.

If you have any concern that the knee or ankle injury
may be serious, go to a doctor. Dr. Kerlan stresses that
there are many tendon and muscle tears that are more
severe than realized, many cracks or breaks in bones that
are not readily recognized, many problem points in the
joints, especially in youngsters, which must be treated
very carefully. For example, there is a point in the lower
front of the knee that sometimes is seriously injured by
youngsters, who shrug off the pain they feel there and
do not go for treatment.

Pulled muscles largely are unavoidable and are treated
initially with pressure ice packs and bandages to control
the swelling and internal bleeding and promote healing.
It must be kept bound tight when not being subjected to
whirlpool baths, and only when it begins to get better
will heat be helpful. As a general rule, it will take 72
hours to heal these sufficiently for a player to resume
heavy activity. Many times it may take longer.

Frank O'Neill points out, "As a trainer for a pro
team, my job, working under a doctor, is to get the players back into action as soon as possible. Everything we
do is directed at this. It is a business and the players'
livelihoods. We will never risk more serious injury to any
athlete, but he is sometimes expected to play uncomfortably.

"It should be obvious, however, that the younger the
player, the lower his level of competition, the less important it be that he be rushed and pushed back into action,
the more important it is that his injury be completely
healed before he takes any chances with it. Youngsters
whose bodies are not fully mature run greater risk of
severe or lingering injuries than do mature pros, and
should be treated accordingly."

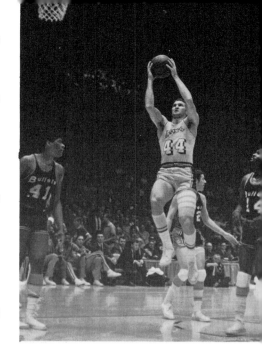

Thigh tightly and heavily bandaged to protect a muscle pull, I go up for a shot against
Baltimore. Looking at this photo, what I
want to know is just what are the Bullets
doing. At the most they're standing around
watching me. One isn't even doing that.
Usually, they're tougher than this. (Photography, Inc.)

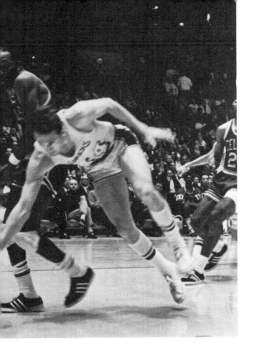

On his way down, "Crash" West may be headed for another ache and pain here. (Photography, Inc.)

"Charley-horses," which really are bruises of the muscles in the thighs or calves should be treated at first with ice- and cold-compresses, then with pressure bandages, later with heat.

Floor burns should be washed with soap and water, dried off, covered with an antiseptic and dressed.

Muscle cramps are nature's way of telling us we are extending some muscles to points of fatigue and exposing them to the dangers of tearing. Often severe sweating—drawing the salt out of the body—contributes to these, and putting salt back into the body helps to stave them off. These may be stretched to points of relief, though this is initially painful. Extend your foot and point your toe as far as possible. In the long run, rest is best, then stretch loose after the pain has passed.

For jammed fingers, guess what? Ice, first. Yes, as a general rule of thumb, freeze injuries, don't fry them. Apply a pressure bandage. Perhaps tape or splint the jammed finger to a fellow finger to give it support.

Again, Dr. Kerlan stresses that in jammed fingers, chipped or broken bones may be overlooked if the finger is not examined by a doctor. To quote Dr. Kerlan, "I really am not one of those who encourages people to run to the doctor with every ache or pain, every bump or bruise. However, in dealing with youngsters engaged in strenuous or rugged games, in youngsters with immature and delicate physical development, some caution must be exercised. If boys eat and sleep sensibly, do not play to the point of exhaustion, do not play when sick or injured, get their sickness and injuries checked and treated, it is not especially dangerous to compete in athletics, and no one should show undue concern about it."

Sometimes it is not injuries that keep a player on the bench. Whatever it is, it is the hardest thing I know to play a game from the bench. Obviously, I have been one of the fortunate ones. I have been a regular, even a star, most of my career. Few are so blessed. However, I was not a starter when I began in school basketball, and I was not even a starter in the first half of my rookie year as pro, though I felt I should have been. My coach, Fred Schaus, thought it would be wiser to bring me along slowly. I didn't (and still don't) agree, but he was the coach and that was that.

Whoever agrees when he isn't playing? Who doesn't think he is better than some of the guys who are in the game? If you don't think you're good enough to play, or at least going to be good enough, you shouldn't be playing. The only reasonable advice anyone can ever give a player in such a situation is that he should keep trying. It doesn't help to moan and groan, to gripe about the coach, and it certainly doesn't help to give up. Keep working in practice, and you may improve enough to become a regular. Many players who are regulars in college and pro ball today were mediocre in earlier days.

Keep up your spirit. Many bench warmers waited a long time to get a shot at a regular job, but became regulars when their chance came, and they were ready to take advantage of it. Many players can make their best contributions as sixth and seventh and eighth men, filling in for the regulars for brief but important stretches. And there are some who simply are not good enough to play regularly who are of real value only in practice. But if you are a member of a team, you owe it to the team to give it whatever it asks of you. A team cannot conduct a full-scale scrimmage with nine men. It needs a tenth man. If you happen to be that man, do your job as best you can.

I'm always unhappy the way many players complain about the coaches behind their backs. Everything is blamed on the coach. Well, there are some bad coaches. But most are equal to their level. And most play the players who will best help them win, because everyone wants to win. Even if a coach has made a mistake where you are concerned, keep trying, bide your time, and

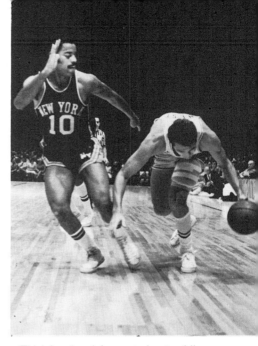

Thigh bandaged, I seem to be stumbling down here under the defensing of Walt Frazier. (Photography, Inc.)

We all sit on the bench sometimes, some of us, sadly, more than others. Here, unhappy at the moment, I sit. (Photography, Inc.)

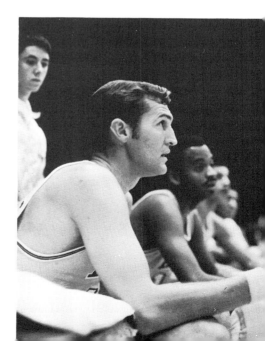

your chance may come. If a person does the best he can, then at least he can hold his head up high.

The team is a fraternity of men, sometimes thrown so closely together it is like a family. When a team stays together, there is a lot of love there. You will not like every player on the team. And you may be jealous of some. And you may resent your coach. But if you pull together you will make the most of every situation.

No one knows what it is to be an athlete except the athlete himself. We are members of a private club and we tend to feel for one another. We know what it is to play and not play, to star or to be benched, to have big nights and bad nights, to work and sacrifice for something and sometimes to get it and sometimes not to get it, to win and to lose. The players on most teams experience a lot together.

In sports we have two families. We have our own families at home. And we have our teams—in the dressing room and on the court, in practice and in games, traveling to and from games together. Respect your coach as you do your parents, and your teammates as you do your brothers and sisters. Give to the team, don't take from it, no matter how hard it may be sometimes. There is a lot to be gained from playing as best we can.

10. In the Clutch

A moment to remember. Here, having stolen the ball on the pass-in to Bob Cousy, I have driven down the court and am just about to lay the ball in for the winning basket as the buzzer sounds in the third game of the 1962 NBA playoff finals. Pursuing me desperately, Cousy just falls short. (UPI)

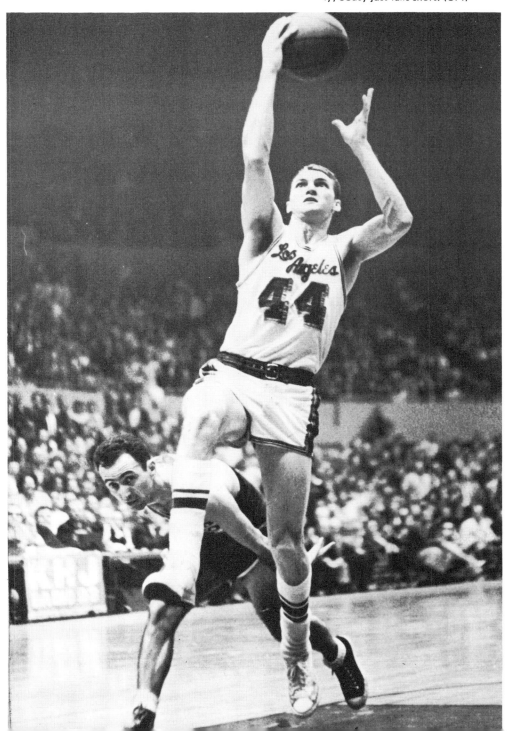

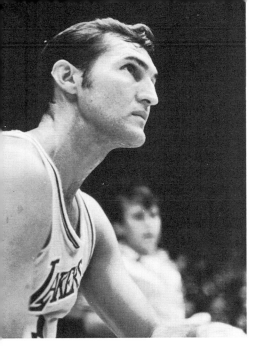

I watch moodily from the sidelines during a moment's rest. I'm not sure it is good to take this game as seriously as I do and maybe I have loosened up a little over the years, but I wouldn't ever want to take it lightly. (Photography, Inc.)

MY NICKNAME and the title of my biography is *Mr. Clutch.* It is embarrassing. When one of my sons asked me what it meant it was difficult to explain it to him without bragging. I certainly never use it and I refer to it here only to make a point. I am proud of it, mind you. Inside, I am quite proud of it. It implies that I come through in the clutch, that I produce under pressure, give the most when it counts the most. What athlete wouldn't be proud of that?

It is not an easy thing to do. The bigger the stakes the harder it is to do your thing. We all feel fear—fear of failure, of losing. The more we want something, the more it means to us, the harder sometimes it is to get it. We all feel a sickness in our gut, a tensing of our muscles in tight times. We all want to be heroes and we're all afraid to be "goats."

I have come through many times in the clutch. On the other hand I have failed, too, in the clutch. And while my team has come close many times, it had never won the NBA playoffs, the world championship, until 1972, which is something I have wanted more than anything else in my athletic life, and I have to hold myself at least partly responsible for this failure. I am a team player. My teams win as teams and lose as teams. We are all responsible. Yet I can't help feeling sometimes I could have done just a little more toward that ultimate triumph.

I hold several NBA playoff records. I had scored more points, 3,708, and averaged more points per game, 30.9, than any player ever through the 1971 playoffs, which I missed with my knee injury. However, this is partly a team triumph, too. I had more opportunity that many great players. With the Lakers I had been in the playoffs ten times, and lasted in them through as many as eighteen games twice. Only Boston Celtic players have had more chances, and they never had a single top scorer.

Aside from the two playoffs I missed entirely or almost entirely, I believe I am the only player ever to average more points in each playoff series than I did in the regular season, until the 1972 playoffs. One year I set a single-season scoring record of 556 points for the playoffs, and the next season I surpassed it with 562. That was in 1969 and 1970, but both seasons wound up with us losing in the seventh game, first to Boston, then to New York.

I suppose my single best playoff came in 1965, however, when Elgin Baylor suffered his crippling knee injury in the first game of the opening series against Baltimore. Picking up a share of the load for Elgin, I scored 49, 52, 44, 48, 43, and 42 points in successive games as we wrapped up the series in six games. But we were in over our heads against Boston in the finals and we lost to them in five games. I scored 43 in one game, 45 in another, but missed 21 out of 27 shots in the last game. I averaged more than 40 points for the entire playoffs, the only player ever to do this.

The 52 was a playoff record for guards, though I surpassed it with 53 in the first game of the finals against Boston in 1969. This is second-best, personally, to my 63, which is a regular-season record for guards, but that was scored in just another game, though one I almost didn't play, as I went into it with a severe cold. It is strange, but sometimes you play your best games when you feel worst, and sometimes you play your worst games when you feel best. All pros will tell you this.

Of course, points are only a part of the overall picture. I think my overall performance—defense, ballhandling, and so forth—improves in the playoffs. I get psyched up for playoffs. It's wrong, but it is a fact that winning a pennant in pro basketball—and pro hockey—is very much secondary to winning the playoffs. All of the glory and most of the money go to those who do best in

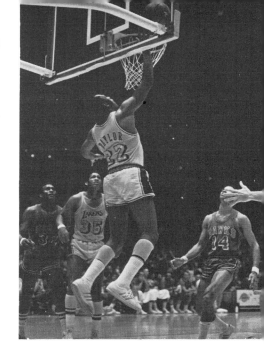

Elgin Baylor whirls in a reverse layup from behind the basket in a playoff against Atlanta. His finest moment under postseason pressure may have come in 1962, when he rejoined the team rusty after army service and in one game against Boston scored a single-game playoff record of 61 points, a mark that still stands. (Photography, Inc.)

the playoffs, so we really spend the long regular season simply preparing for the playoffs, trying to get the best possible position for the playoffs, and the real season is the second season, the short season of the playoffs.

I always have tried harder in playoffs, but the only other real championship I have helped with in my life other than the 1972 NBA Championship was the West Virginia High School tournament title with my East Bank team in my senior year, 1956. Along the way we almost lost out in the regional finals against Nitro, a school we had beaten easily during the regular season. It may be we were overconfident. At one point, Nitro scored 17 straight points and they had us at halftime by 17. We were sick and sorry youngsters in the dressing room. Seventeen points is a tremendous lead in high school play. The halves are short and players seldom have the poise to make up that much of a deficit.

I learned something that night—that you never know when you can turn a seemingly impossible situation around, that if you give your best no matter the odds against you, once in a while you will swing a tremendous upset. We began to chase Nitro all over the court. We scored while they didn't score a basket for five minutes. We began to close in and by the end of three periods, we were within 9 points. Then they tried to freeze the ball and fell completely apart. We caught 'em and passed 'em, and I was dribbling the ball at the final buzzer protecting a 70-65 lead and threw the ball high in the air, and we mobbed one another.

In the next-to-last game we were behind by as much as 11 points in the last quarter and five in the last few minutes, but we'd learned our lesson and we kept trying. I got the ball and sank a layup to cut it to 3. I got it again and sank a jumper and we were within 1, and that fieldhouse was a madhouse. They had the ball but I tied up my man, forcing a jump. Our coach, Roy Williams, called a time-out and told me to slap the ball as far

downcourt as I could on the jump and told Jack
Landers, a teammate, to break downcourt the minute
the ball was thrown up. I had to win the jump. I did, and
slapped it downcourt. Landers grabbed it on his way to
the basket and laid it in and the buzzer went off and we
had won, 64-63. All was madness again.

The key plays in that game were tying a man up and
winning a jump. Details. Coming from behind. Staying
cool. If something is working for you, stay with it. I am
against successfully building a lead, then shifting styles
and sitting on it. Perhaps you get a bit more conservative
with a lead to protect, but never leave something that is
successful for you. Very often when, say, a freeze fails
and you try to go back to running, you find that you
have lost your rhythm and can't swing it. More than
anything else, I believe you should never give up. That
may be a cliché, but I mean it.

No matter what the situation in a given game, give
your best every minute of every game. Work on it, concentrate on it. When you are 10 or 20 points ahead, or
far ahead in a pennant race, it is very hard not to feel
like a winner, not to ease off and look ahead to the rewards of your success. But just blow a big game or a
pennant once because you were coasting and you'll remember it for a long time, perhaps forever. And I hate
to think of the teams in basketball, football, hockey,
and baseball that have gone into losing streaks and
blown "sure" crowns in the stretch. And I also hate to
think of the teams that got discouraged and tailed off
and said, "Hey, the team that won was really faltering at
the finish. If we'd done just a little more here and a little
more there, we still could have taken them." It is a terrible feeling.

Play every game as it comes up, one game at a time.
More than that, play 'em one play at a time. Never look
beyond right now. Never underestimate any foe. Bad
teams are easier to beat than good teams, but losses to

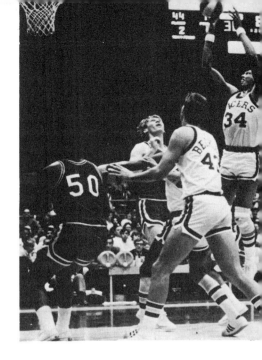

Mel Daniels (34), star center of Bobby
Leonard's Indiana Pacers, pops in a bucket
during that team's pressure-packed run to
the 1970 ABA playoff title. In 1971 the
Pacers were dethroned by Bill Sharman's
Utah Stars in another clutch playoff. Whether in the NBA or ABA, the team that takes
the tension best and wins the title is to be
saluted. (Indiana Pacers)

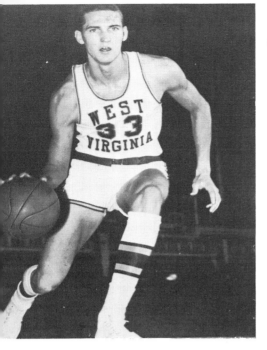

A young Jerry West at West Virginia University. (WVU Photo)

bad teams hurt more than those to good teams. If you are a good team, you're going to lose some to other good teams, but you shouldn't lose many to bad teams. Losses to bad teams cost many teams titles. And there is hardly a league in the country where the bad team isn't good enough to beat the good team if the good team plays badly. It is that simple. Respect all your opponents. The game isn't won until you're back home with the victory. The title isn't won until the season ends.

Look at it this way: Play with pride. Give your best in all situations. Some situations may turn out really hopeless. Sometimes you are eliminated from a pennant race early. But you should always do the best you possibly can, individually, and you always want to help your team do the best it can, collectively. Some say that after first place, all other places are nowhere. To some degree, I feel this, too. But second place is really better than third. And in pro ball, fourth place gets you into the playoffs and gives you a chance to win it all. In any event, always be able to walk away from a game or a season with your head held high, knowing you did your best right down to last place. And there will be times you will be rewarded with surprising success.

You will not always win. At West Virginia University, in my sophomore season, we went into the first round of the NCAA playoffs with a 26-1 record and a fine chance of going all the way, but we lost the first game by 5 points to a weak Manhattan team we should have beaten by 20 points. And if we had played them the following night we would have. If we had played them a hundred times we'd have beaten them 99 times. But this was the hundredth time.

The following season we went all the way to the final game. Along the way we trailed St. Joseph's of Philadelphia by 18 points with 13 minutes left. Schaus moved me into the pivot and I scored 14 points in less than 4 minutes. With 1 minute to go we were within a point of

them and we stole the ball and I drove in for a layup
that put us ahead. When I got the ball again I got fouled
and sank the two free-throws to sew it up. By the final
game, against Darrall Imhoff's University of California
team, a late rally fell short and we lost by a point. I had
the ball in my hands and was ready to go for the winning
basket when the buzzer went off. I didn't even get the
shot off. It was a terrible disappointment.

My senior season we were upset by NYU early in the
NCAA tournament and that was it. You only get a few
chances to go for the college crown and, unless you go
to UCLA, you don't win many. If you are on a team
that has a good shot at the title, it is a terrible disappointment and stays with you forever. I had one consolation that year in that I got to play on the U.S. Olympic
team that won the gold medal in basketball in Rome. On
that team were such players as Oscar Robertson, Jerry
Lucas, Darrall Imhoff, Walt Bellamy, Bob Boozer, and
Adrian Smith.

The 1958 Olympic championship U.S.A.
team. In the front row are the coaches, including head coach Pete Newell, right. In
the second row are Les Lane, Al Kelly, Adrian Smith, Jay Armette, me, and the trainer. In the third row are Darrall Imhoff, Jerry
Lucas, Walt Bellamy, Burdie Haldersen, Bob
Boozer, Terry Dischinger, and Oscar Robertson.

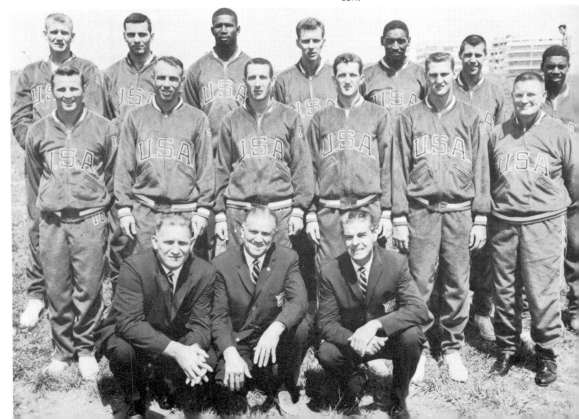

In my first ten years with the Lakers, we won six
divisional pennants and won seven divisional playoffs,
but lost in the finals every time, four times in the
seventh and final game, once in overtime, twice by 2
points, once by 3 points. Put that way, statistically, it is
sad, but not overwhelming. However, year after year,
blow after blow, going to the wire so often and always
falling short, it was frankly almost too much to bear.
Elgin and I were the only Lakers who endured that
whole stretch, although Fred Schaus was either coach or
general manager throughout.

There have been other high and low points for me
personally. In my first playoff finals against Boston in
1962, my second season in the NBA, I missed 17 of 22
shots in the first game. We lost it but won the second
game and came home for the third game all even. With a
minute or so to play, they had us by 4. I got the ball,
jumped, shot, and hit. They brought the ball back and
missed a shot. I got the ball, jumped, and again hit, tie-
ing the game as the Sports Arena fans went wild.

The Celtics had the ball and called time-out with just
3 seconds left and set up a last play. Sam Jones took the
ball out and I was guarding Bob Cousy, who was to be
their ballhandler, I figured. I laid off him a little, but as
Sam's hands began to move I began to move. As the ball
was thrown toward Cousy I jumped in front of him and
grabbed it, pushed it in front of me, and followed it.
Dribbling, afraid the buzzer would go off, I pulled the
ball up, jumped, leaned toward the backboard and laid
the ball in. As it was going through the cords the buzzer
sounded. We had won.

It was a moment of madness. I remember lying in bed
and thinking about it. We all want to hit a home run in
the ninth to win a game in the World Series. That was
my home run. Not many fellows ever have such a moment in their lives, I suppose, and I'll never forget it.
That moment is my trophy and I wish I could bronze it.

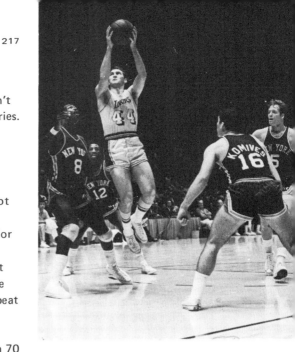

Here I lay one up against a New York Knick team of a few years ago. Knicks are Walt Bellamy, Dick Barnett, Howie Komives, and Dick Van Arsdale. (Photography, Inc.)

The story has a sad ending, however. The war wasn't over. We lost the next game, falling back to an even series. We won in Boston, however, and came home with a chance to wrap it up. We led by 8 at halftime of the sixth game. I suppose we counted on it before it was won. I was tired and didn't work for shots and didn't shoot much in the third quarter. We stood around a lot and they caught us and beat us bad. In Boston in the seventh game we traded the lead back and forth. Baylor scored 41 points in that game. We were tied with 18 seconds left and had the last shot. Frank Selvy took it with 3 seconds left. It was a short, open shot from the side and he hit the rim with it and it went off. They beat us in overtime. Russell wound up with 40 rebounds.

The next season we were playing St. Louis in the playoffs and they led us in one game by 7 points with 70 seconds to play. I hit two baskets and we caught up with 7 seconds to go, but the Hawks had the ball and were playing for the last shot. Cliff Hagan was dribbling and he wasn't my man, so he wasn't looking for me, but I dropped off my man, dove and knocked the ball away, stumbled right over him, got the ball, drove with it, grabbed it at the free-throw line, and shot a jumper, which went through as the buzzer went off. This was a great moment, too. We won the series in seven games, but lost the finals.

In 1966 we lost three of the first four games of the finals, but then won two straight to tie it before we lost the last one. We came from 10 points to 2 points behind in the last few minutes, but we didn't come back any further. That was the eighth-straight NBA title for Boston under Red Auerbach's coaching.

In 1968 Bill Russell was coaching and playing, but he was getting old, and the whole Celtic team was tired, and we may have been a better team by then, and we should have beaten them—but we didn't. In the last few minutes of a game that was already lost, the fourth game, I dove

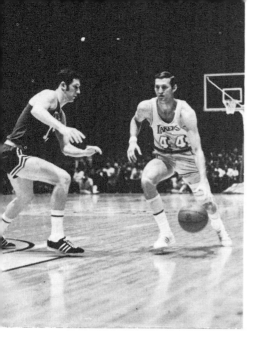

I dribble-drive on John Havlicek in one of those L.A.-Boston playoff series. I gained series MVP honors, but I must say Havlicek is an incredible competitor who played full games tirelessly and had a sensational series when the Celtics won the one they should not have won from us in 1969. Usually, they were the better team and should have won, which does not mean we could not have upset them, but in 1969 we should have won, which made it the one that hurt the most. (Photography, Inc.)

for a loose ball, collided with John Havlicek, and went down heavily, spraining my left ankle severely. I'll never regret trying to make the play, but it was a costly one. I was handicapped for the rest of the series.

In the fifth game we trailed by 19, but we kept coming and with 12 seconds left I put in a layup to tie it. They lost the ball and we had a chance to win, but Elg barely missed an off-balance shot he had to try with time running out, and they won in overtime and went on to win in six games.

In 1969 the Celtics barely made it into the playoffs and we definitely were the better team—except that they were, because they won. We had Wilt then. I shot more than usual in the first game, 41 times, because the openings were there, and scored 53 and we won. And we won the second, but I fell and banged my right hand and it was swollen and sore after that, though it didn't bother me too much. They won two in Boston, the last one on a crazy off-balance shot by Sam Jones, to even the series.

We won the fifth, but I pulled a hamstring muscle in my left leg and it hurt the rest of the way. We lost the sixth there. And we came home and lost the seventh. I remember I lost the ball on a key play late when I dribbled the ball off Em Bryant's knee. We lost by 2 points. I'd had a super-scoring series and *Sport* magazine gave me the new car they give to the MVP in the playoff finals, a rare honor for a loser, but I was a loser and it was at best a consolation prize.

All those years it was the Boston Celtics who beat us in the finals, but after Bill Russell retired it was the New York Knicks who took us. Wilt hurt his knee and was out most of the season, but he got back by the playoffs, and again we had a good chance. I bruised my right hand badly during the playoffs. However, you can't take time off during the playoffs.

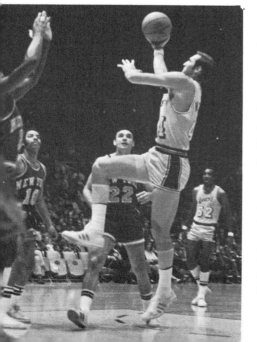

We had a good shot at it in 1970, too, against New York, and should have won after Willis Reed was hurt, but did not. Here I shoot over Willis Reed while Walt Frazier and Dave DeBusschere watch. I surpassed the playoff scoring record I'd set the year before, but it was still another loss. (Photography, Inc.)

We split the first two games and were behind by 2
points with seconds left in the third game. We had the
ball out at our end, but no time really to do anything.
The pass was hurriedly thrown in to me. I was on my
side of the midcourt line, but I knew I had to shoot, so I
just pushed up a one-hander with all my might, and it's
funny, but as it was going I really thought it would go
in, and it did, and there was a split-second of silence and
then a tremendous explosion of noise.

I figure it was about a 60-foot shot, but it has been
measured at 63 feet, and there is a marker on the Forum
floor now memoralizing the place from which I shot. It
has been called "the most incredible shot," and it certainly was my most remarkable, but I just shot it, and it
just went in and I've never tried another like it since,
even in practice.

The sad thing is that everyone was dancing around
and screaming, and most thought the game was over. But
it wasn't, it only tied the game. Wilt even started to run
off the court and had to return in embarrassment. And
then we lost in overtime. So what was it? The shot
meant nothing. Afterward, when everyone was asking
me excitedly about the shot, I had to keep reminding
them that we'd lost the game. I finally went off to hide.
I wanted to cry. It was spoiled. I'm proud of the shot
and will remember it forever, but I'd rather have won
than shot it. You win or you lose, that's what counts.

When Willis Reed, the key Knick, got hurt in the
fifth game, we built a big lead and should have won easily, but we fell apart while they pulled together and they
caught us and beat us. Without Willis, the Knicks were
routed in the sixth game, but then we had to go back to
New York for the seventh game, and with our history it
was hard to believe we'd win. And we didn't, even
though Willis was only limping around by then. They
shot hot, built a big lead, and held on to it easily.

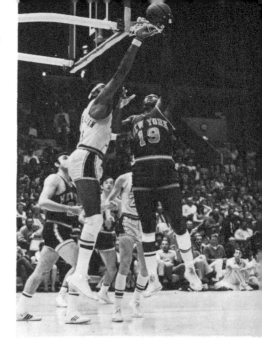

Outstanding clutch showings were made in
the 1970 playoffs by Willis Reed (above)
laying one in over Wilt Chamberlain, and
Dick Barnett (below) popping one in over
Dick Garrett. Reed performed in the latter
part in pain while Frazier was spectacular in
the final game. (Photography, Inc.)

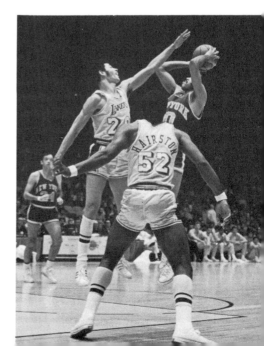

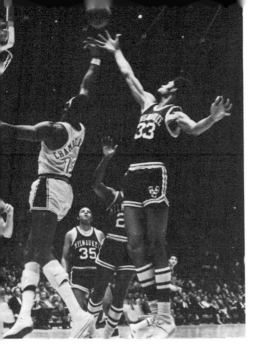

Brilliant performances under pressure in the
1971 playoffs were given by Milwaukee's
Jabbar (above), vying for a rebound with
Wilt Chamberlain, and Oscar Robertson
(below) eluding Keith Erickson around a
screen by Connie Dierking in an earlier day.
Oscar never had a real good chance while
with the Royals but showed his class in the
clutch with the Bucks. (Photography, Inc.)

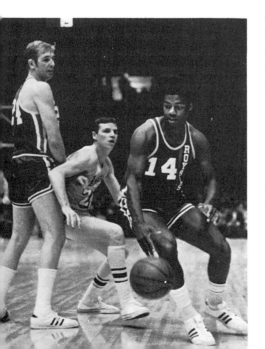

I think maybe we felt we were jinxed, maybe we
didn't go into the game with enough confidence. Without Willis they weren't as good as we were, even with the
home-court edge. The home-court edge is mostly psychological. A fellow should play as well on the road as at
home. Maybe if we could have forgotten the past we
would have won in the present.

I was hurt and out of the playoffs in 1971, and Willis
was hurt again and Kareem Abdul-Jabbar and Oscar
Robertson led Milwaukee to the title. Reed had proven
himself as a pressure player the year before, and then
Jabbar proved himself as a pro, though he certainly had
established his clutch instincts by leading UCLA to
three-straight NCAA titles before he turned pro.

However, I really believe Robertson was the outstanding performer in the 1971 finals. Perhaps there's some
sentiment behind this. Like me, he'd never played on a
championship team. Actually, his Cincinnati club seldom
was even a strong contender. But when he got with a
strong Milwaukee club, even with a sore leg he was masterful, quarterbacking the team, orchestrating the games,
making the big plays, seldom shooting, but making good
shots, proving himself under pressure and helping his
team take the title I always wanted so much, and I'm
sure he wanted just as much.

The 1971-72 season was an exceptional one for me,
which makes me look forward to the 1972-73 season.
Bill Sharman came in as coach and converted us to a
running game and a style of team play which paid divi-
dends. Our streak of 33 straight victories, unsurpassed in
professional team sports, was a tremendous experience.
It was not easy to sustain this, but we did, through two
full calendar months.

Elgin Baylor had just retired, Wilt Chamberlain had
just taken over as team captain, and I had just come off
the injured list, and I was not to miss another game all
season. Happy Hairston joined Wilt in a great rebounding
effort, and Jim McMillian joined Gail Goodrich in a great

shooting effort. Pat Riley, Leroy Ellis, John Q. Trapp,
Flynn Robinson and others came off the bench to contribute. Even after the streak was over, we avoided any
prolonged letdown or slump. We were able to adjust to
any game and win regularly on the road as well as at
home.

We finished with 69 victories and only 13 defeats, the
best record in the history of the NBA. Many felt Wilt
was the Most Valuable Player in the league. As it turned
out, I finished second in the voting to Jabbar for the
third straight season, just ahead of Wilt, and while I
would have loved to have won once, and would have
understood Wilt winning again, I could not complain
about Jabbar winning. These things are not that important.

I did win the MVP Trophy in the mid-season All-Star
Game, which was a big thrill, especially as it was played
in our Forum and before my wife and sons. I stole the
ball a number of times, scored well and scored the last-
second shot that brought West the victory. However,
individual awards and winning streaks are secondary
things next to the team championship.

In 1972, we had a splendid series in eliminating Chicago with four straight victories in the first round, then
struggled to the Western Division title by dethroning
Jabbar and his Milwaukee Bucks in six games in a see-
saw series which started with us being routed at home
and wound up with us rallying to beat them on the road.
Oscar Robertson was handicapped with an injury, but
we have been handicapped with key injuries in past playoffs. So we reached the finals for the eighth time in my
12 years as a pro.

New York had an ordinary season, but had made
adjustments to new players such as Earl Monroe and
Jerry Lucas, who filled in at center for the injured Willis
Reed, and were coming fast at the finish. Injuries to
Dick Barnett and then Dave DeBusschere handicapped
them, but they had great balance, great discipline, great

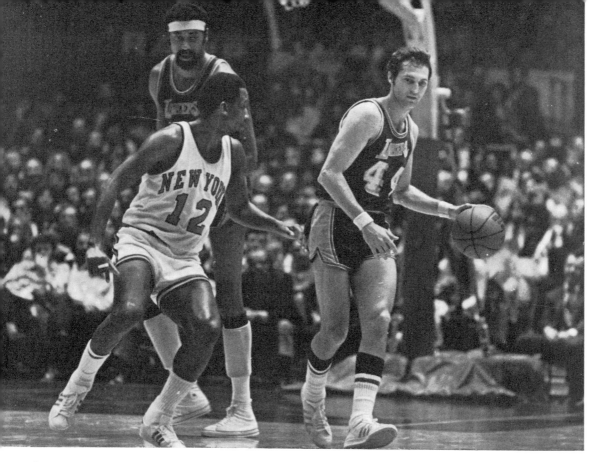

On the way to the championship at last, I dribble against Dick Barnett of the Knicks while my Laker teammate Wilt Chamberlain, who had such a sensational series and was MVP winner of the car awarded by *Sport* magazine, looks on. Gail Goodrich also had a great series, as did Jim McMillian, Happy Hairston, Pat Riley, Leroy Ellis and the rest. And Bill Sharman's coaching made the difference for us. He stressed sacrifice, conditioning, team play and a running style which really paid off. (Photography, Inc.)

coaching from Red Holzman and some of the best outside shooters I've ever seen on one team. Lucas, DeBusschere, Bradley, Frazier, Monroe and reserves Dean Meminger and Phil Jackson formed a fine team, as strong in its way as the 1970 championship Knicks were.

Beating them and finally capturing the championship after those seemingly endless seasons of disappointment had to be the greatest thrill of my career, although I suffered through a shooting slump. I was able to contribute in a variety of ways, as were our other players. I'm not sure if this one wipes out all the others, but after struggling through all those years of pressure playoffs, it sure was something to be on the winning side at last.

Some of the best players in basketball are not at their

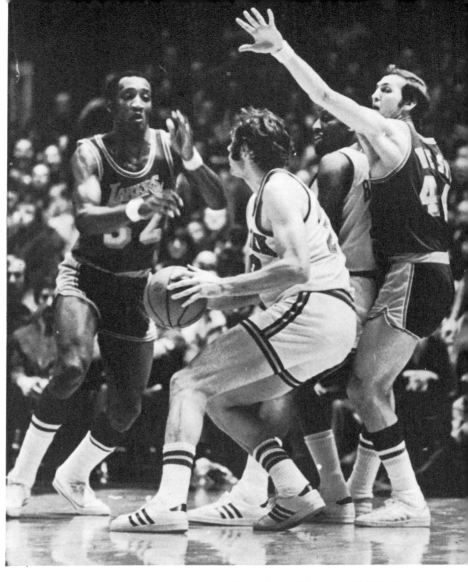

best under pressure. Even pros are human. I've seen players' shorts quivering, their rear-end muscles shaking from nerves in tight moments. Some of them don't want the ball in the clutch. I do. I feel I am doing something good with it. The fact is, I can't always, and often haven't. But I have done it enough to have confidence in my ability to do it.

All players should think that way. I think they should

Here, Happy Hairston and I defend on Dave DeBusschere, who, with Jerry Lucas, Bill Bradley, Walt Frazier and other Knicks, gave us plenty of trouble in the NBA playoff finals in 1972, which ended with my Lakers winning the title that had eluded us so long. Dave had an injured side, but Happy had an injured foot. You play with injuries, especially in playoffs. Wilt played in the final game with bad hands and wrists. Winning it all was a fantastic feeling. (Photography, Inc.)

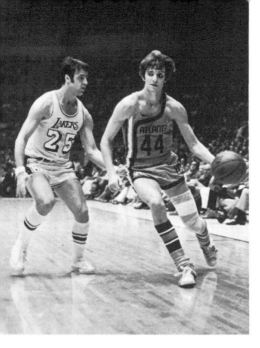

Gail Goodrich, here guarding Pete Maravich, really showed me a lot by the way he took the tension and stole the show as the Lakers upset Chicago in the first round of the 1971 playoffs with me out before falling to a favored Milwaukee team. Maravich, whose college teams won no titles, must learn to take playoff pressure. (Photography, Inc.)

The big man, Bill Russell, hauling down a rebound in the playoffs. (Photography, Inc.)

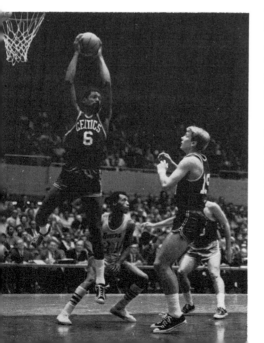

build up their abilities to the highest level they can and build up their confidence. They should welcome the opportunity to do the things they do best when it counts the most.

You have to concentrate on the play. You can't be thinking about how much it means. If you are going to be a player on a team, you have to accept, even welcome, responsibility. That doesn't mean you should take the shot away from your team's best shooter, but it means you should want to play your part under pressure. You have to fight fear.

Maybe some of it is ego, but you have to have a controlled ego to play this game right. If a fellow embarrasses you on a given play, you can't try to get back at him on every play the rest of the game. You have to try to beat him when it's the situation for you to go against him. You have to let it go and pass-off or work on someone else when the situation calls for it. You have to have confidence and pride, but you can't let it get in the way of playing for the team.

I've known many outstanding clutch players in basketball, and I'd have to say that Bill Russell was the one I admired the most, because his teams won the most. He was not the only fine pressure player on his teams. Certainly, John Havlicek and Sam Jones and others were fantastic competitors in the clutch, but Bill was the big man. He wasn't a big scorer, but he got the baskets his team needed, he got the rebounds his team needed, he made the plays they needed, he did the defensive job, he blocked the shots, he ran the show, he inspired his team. It's on the record what his team did with him, and what it did before him, and after him.

There is some pressure in every game. Certainly, as the young player moves up, the pressure on him increases. It is hard to play before crowds at first, then before big crowds in big arenas. It is hard to play for titles. It is not easy to be a player in any sport. I think

that if you clear your mind of all other thoughts before
a game and concentrate only on the game while you are
playing it, and if you take it one play at a time, always
giving your all, it will become a way of life for you.

You can't be up for every game, but you can try to
be. If you are intense, you will lose your temper during
games, but you can try to control yourself. If you make
a mistake, you will get angry with yourself, but you can
try not to make the same mistake the next time. You
can put it away and go on to the next play. Griping to
the refs comes easy, but gets you nowhere. They have a
tough job to do, too, maybe the toughest in sports. Try
to control your emotions.

There are players who have the ability to play a game
on the top level who don't care about the game all that
much, or are lazy or more interested in having fun away
from the game, but these are not good examples to follow. Whatever you are doing, you should do it as best
you can. For me fun on a basketball court means trying
to do well and win games, but this is a very serious sort
of fun, so I'll let the parties and the golf and the fishing
wait. I think in games you should always give that good
second-effort and even third-effort, because this is what
separates most good players from most ordinary players,
and it is what wins most games. Always be able to walk
away with your head held high.

Try to treat everyone as you want to be treated. If
you don't like someone, do with him only what you
have to do with him, but do it right, for if he is your
teammate, you and he are responsible to one another
and to the team. Don't be a pop-off or a clubhouse law-
yer. Hold your hard thoughts in and try to proceed with
dignity. Give 100 percent if possible. Not "110" percent. In the end we'll get our just due. People are
amazed that Elgin Baylor and I have been able to share
"superstardom" all these years. There's nothing amazing
about it. We respect each other. I'm proud that we've

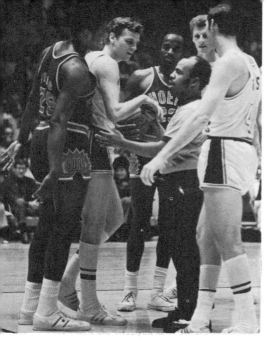

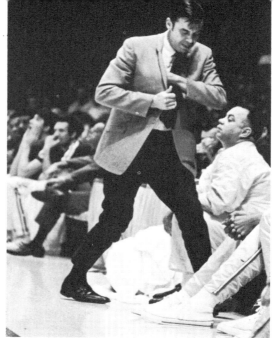

Tempers flare in tense action. Above left, Keith Erickson gives the smallest ref, Ken Hudson, a piece of his mind while Paul Silas, Art Harris, Mel Counts, and yours truly crowd around. Above right, coach Bill van Breda Kolff storms on the sidelines. Below, Toby Kimball (7) and Elvin Hayes argue in amazement with ref Darell Garretson. (Photography, Inc.)

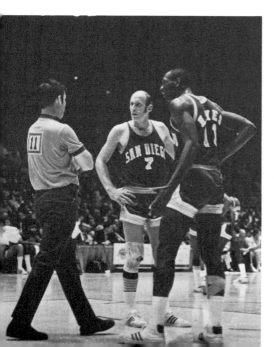

worked together in harmony for all our careers. And it hasn't cost either of us a thing. We've gained from it.

I've known guys who didn't put out all the time, who paled under pressure, who were able to clown around in the locker room after a serious loss. I don't respect them, but I've learned to live with them, so I just do my best and let the others do their thing, and I try to keep my respect for myself. Discipline yourself and have respect for authority. Try for modesty. Don't be carried away with yourself. I guarantee you there's always someone better.

I feel that all the years I put into basketball, learning the game and growing up in it, have paid me fantastic rewards, and I am deeply grateful. In sports, players ride a rollercoaster of emotions. They get very high and very low. You have to learn to handle this, to keep everything in the right perspective. Win or lose, there probably will be another time.

For me, it has all been worthwhile. I have a fine family and lead a good life. I have a good name and I have accomplished a lot in my profession. I think the boy who starts playing basketball should begin as if it were going to be a big thing to him. I can't compare playing a game well to researching a cure for a disease or other praiseworthy pursuits, but athletics can be an admirable way to earn a livelihood, and the beginner may embark on a career when he is least expecting it. Anyway, as long as he is doing it, he should try to do it right.

I have tried to tell you my way, which is that there are many ways. I hope I have helped you to find your own way.

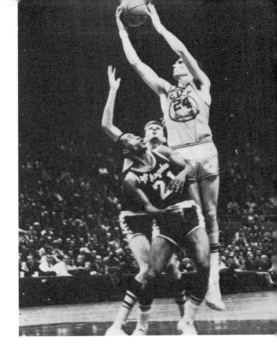

Rick Barry, an intense player who is given to emotional outbursts, nevertheless seems at his best under playoff pressure and has given brilliant performances in postseason play both in the NBA and ABA. In the 1971 ABA playoffs, though not normally an outside shooter, he set a record for 3-point shooting. He gets psyched up. (San Francisco Warriors)

Driving on Larry Siegfried, Bill Russell waits on me in one of those memorable Celtic-Laker playoffs. (Photography, Inc.)

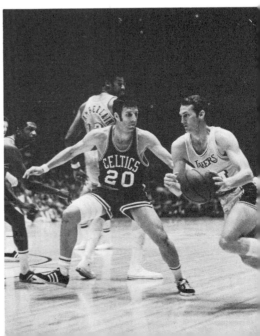

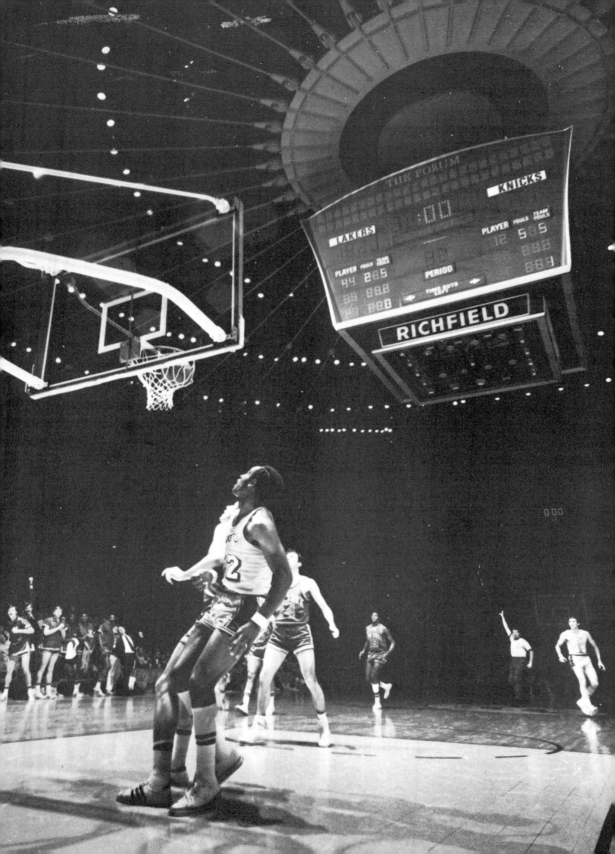

The 63-foot shot that tied the third game of the NBA playoff finals of 1970 against New York. There is no time showing on the scoreboard as the shot is going through the hoop in this dramatic photo. I am at the rear right, watching from the point at which I released the ball. The ref has his arm in the air indicating that time ran out while the ball was in flight. Happy Hairston and a Knick are waiting under the bucket and everyone else is watching expectantly. Jack Kent Cooke's Forum exploded seconds later, but the sad end came when the Knicks won the game in overtime. I do not teach this shot. (Sheedy & Long for *Sports Illustrated* © Time, Inc.)

A Portfolio of the Playoffs

The Lakers' '72 Title Drive

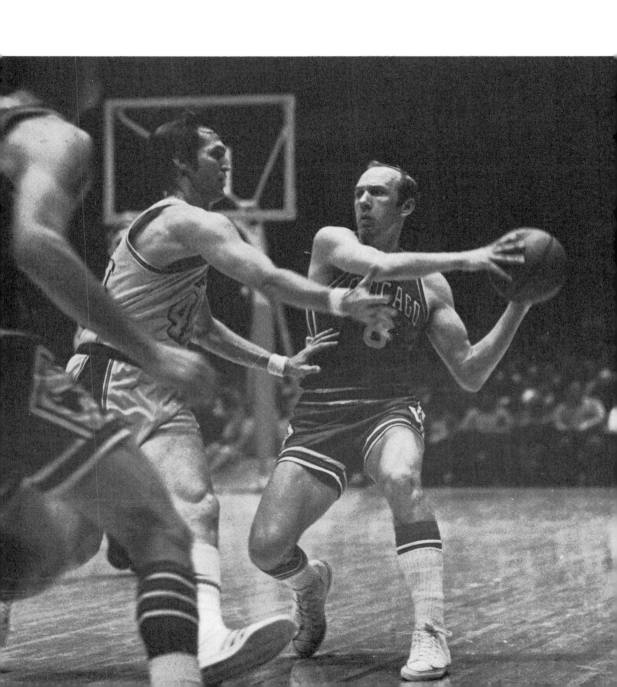

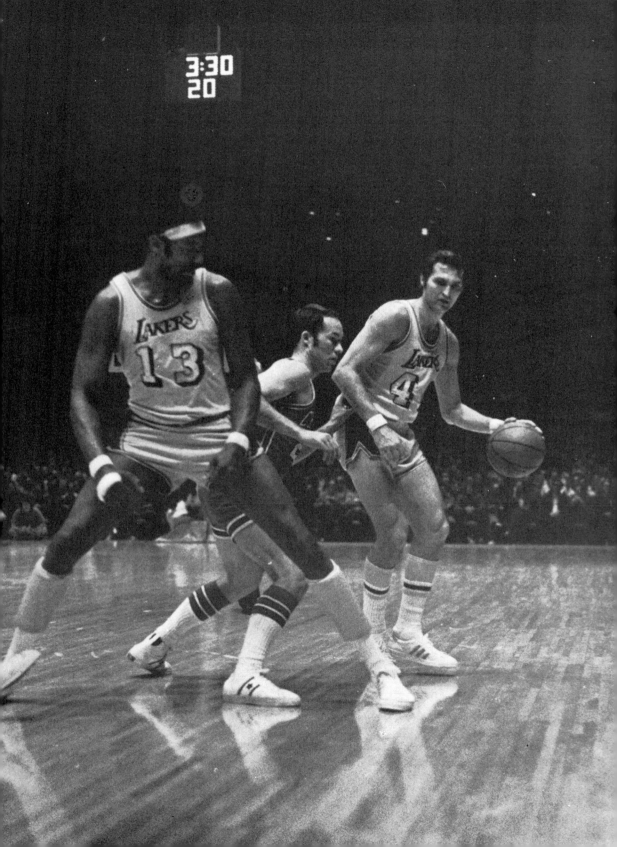

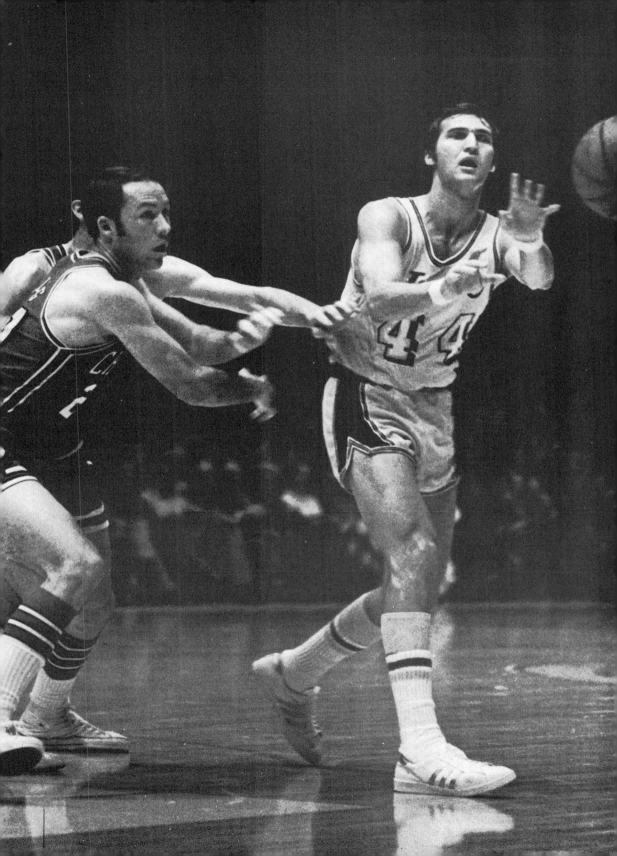

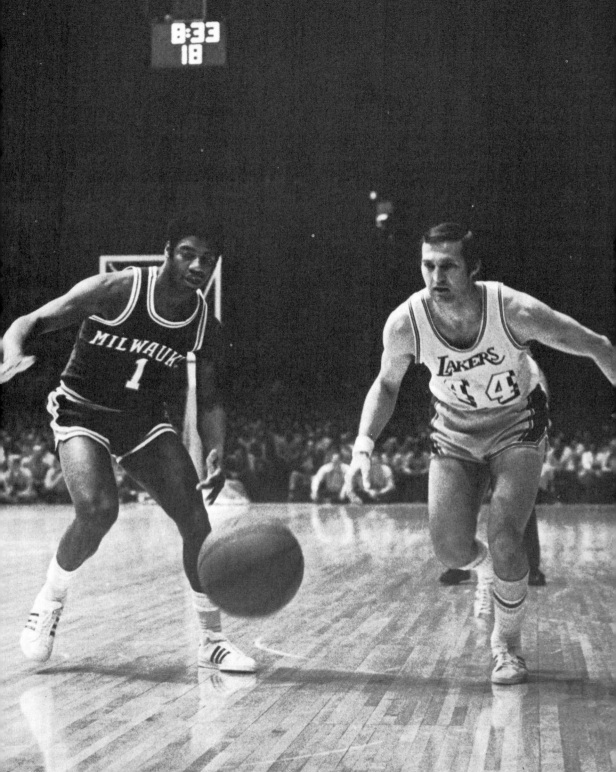

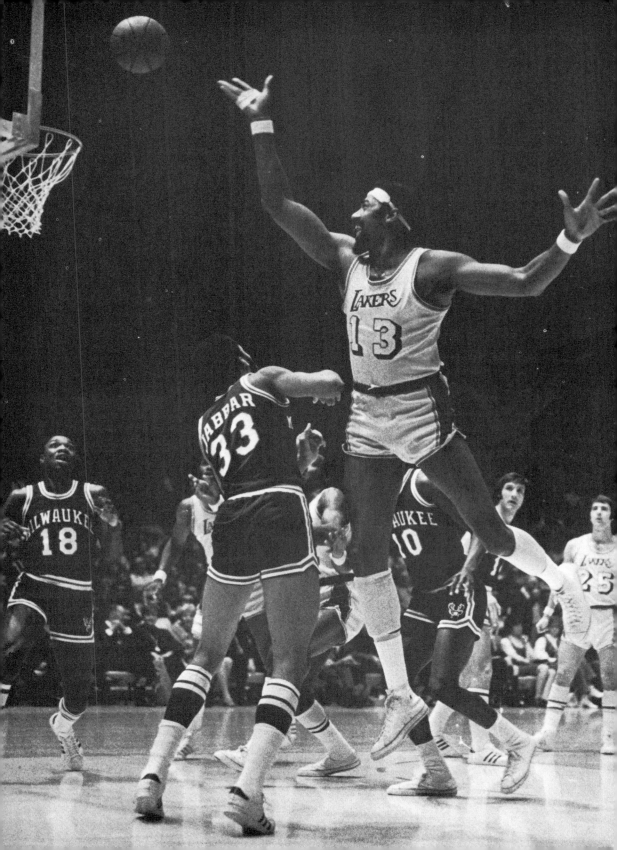

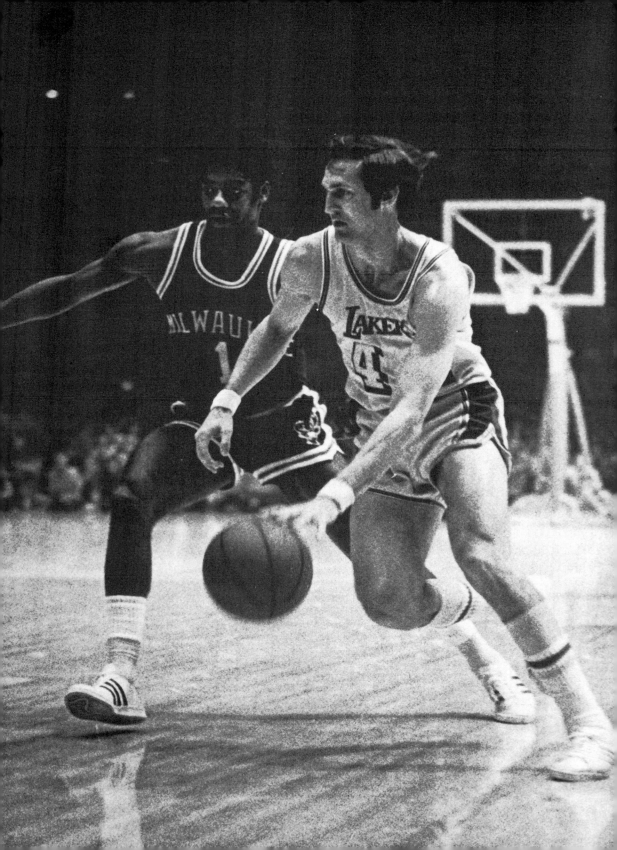

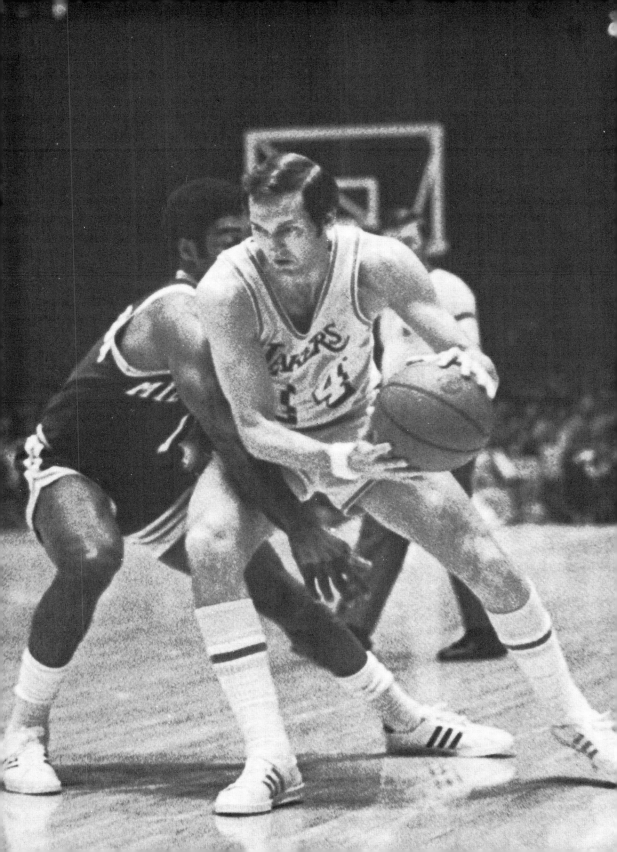

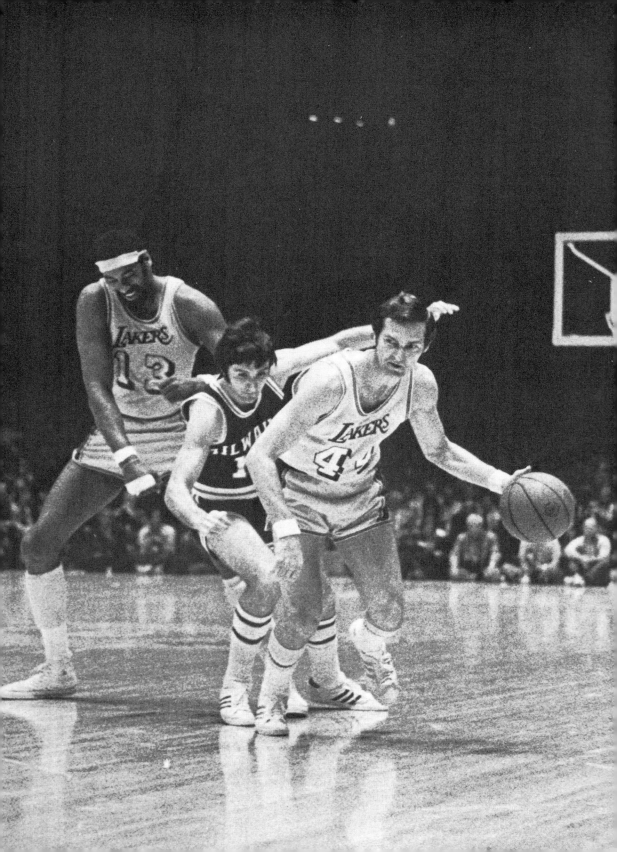

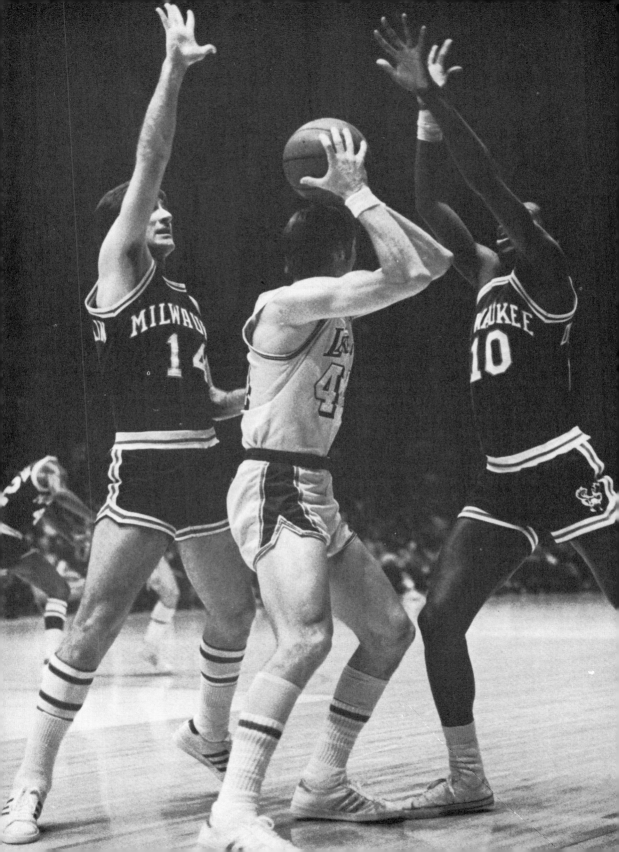

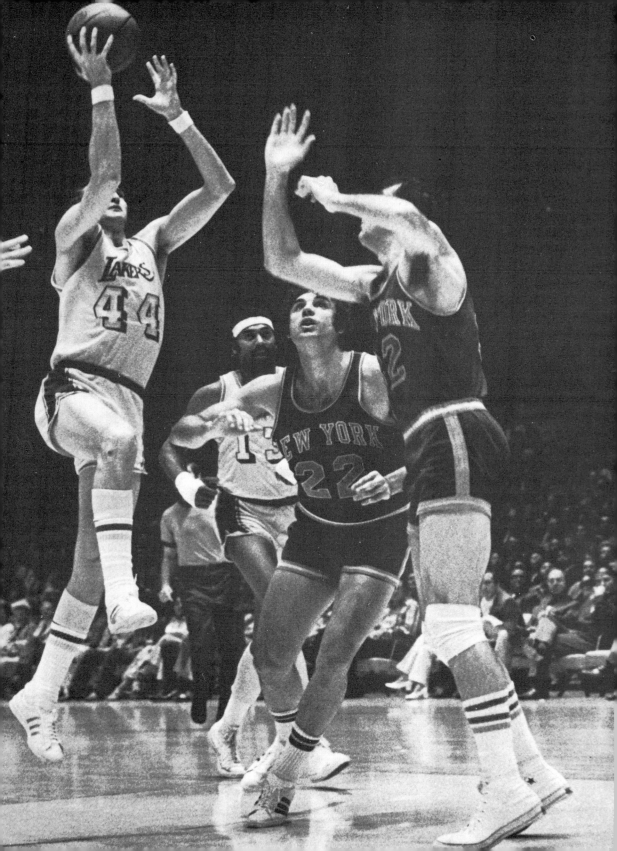

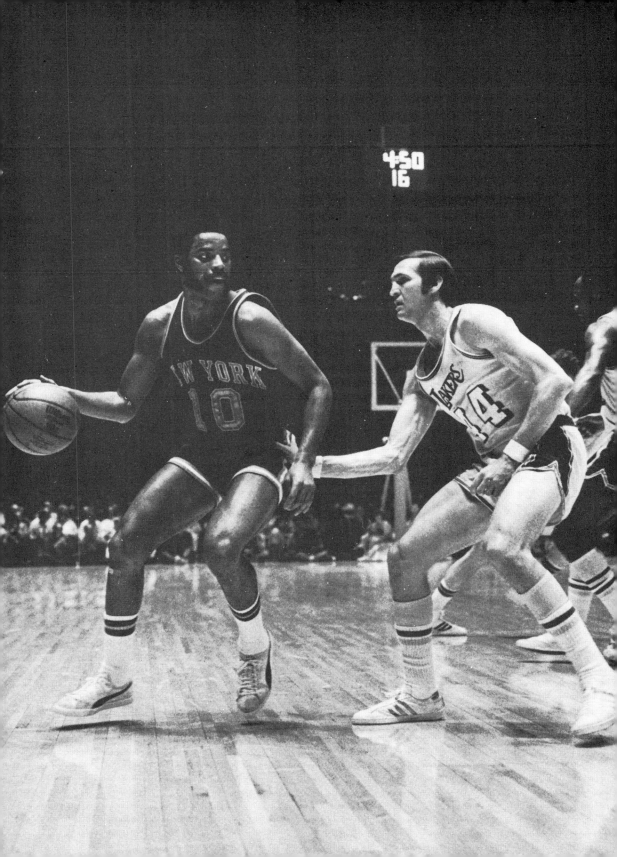

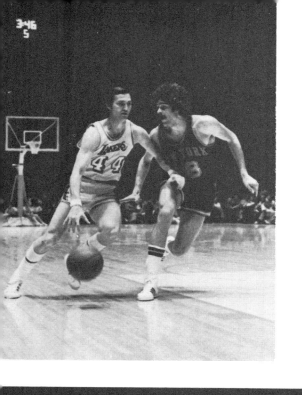

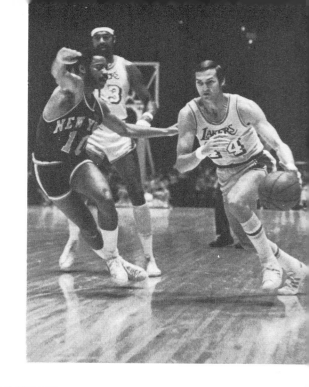

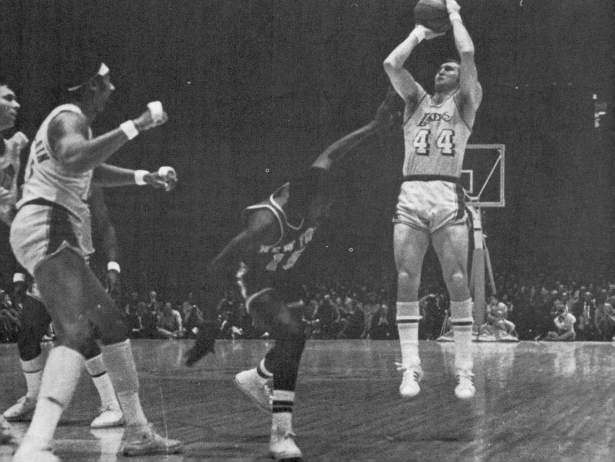